Neoplasms
of the Colon, Rectum,
and Anus

Neoplasms
of the Colon, Rectum,
and Anus

Edited by

MAUS W. STEARNS, JR., M.D.

Former Chief, Rectum and Colon Service
Memorial Sloan-Kettering Cancer Center
New York, New York

A WILEY MEDICAL PUBLICATION
JOHN WILEY & SONS
New York • Chichester • Brisbane • Toronto

Library of Congress Cataloging in Publication Data:

Main entry under title:

Neoplasms of the colon, rectum, and anus.

  (A Wiley medical publication)
  Includes index.
  1. Colon (Anatomy)—Cancer. 2. Rectum—
Cancer. 3. Anus—Cancer. I. Stearns, Maus W.
[DNLM: 1. Anus neoplasms. 2. Colonic neoplasms.
3. Rectal neoplasms. WI610 N438]
RC280.C6N46   616.99'2347   79-29671
ISBN 0-471-05924-2

Printed in the United States of America

10 9 8 7 6 5 4 3 2 1

This book is dedicated to those patients whose disease provided the experience reflected in this review

Contributors

Fadi F. Attiyeh, M.D.
Assistant Attending Surgeon
Rectum and Colon Service
Memorial Sloan-Kettering Cancer Center
New York, New York

Robert Golbey, M.D.
Chief of Solid Tumor Service
Department of Medicine
Memorial Sloan-Kettering Cancer Center
New York, New York

Ralph E. L. Hertz, M.D.
New York, New York

Nancy Kemeny, M.D.
Assistant Attending Physician
Solid Tumor Service
Department of Medicine
Memorial Sloan-Kettering Cancer Center
New York, New York

Charles S. LaMonte, M.D.
Acting Chief, Cardiopulmonary Service
Department of Medicine
Memorial Hospital for Cancer and Allied Diseases
New York, New York

Robert Leaming, M.D.
Assistant Attending Radiation Therapist
Radiation Therapy Department
Memorial Sloan-Kettering Cancer Center
New York, New York

Stuart H. Q. Quan, M.D.
Attending Surgeon
Rectum and Colon Service
Memorial Sloan-Kettering Cancer Center
New York, New York

Paul Sherlock, M.D.
Chairman, Department of Medicine
Memorial Sloan-Kettering Cancer Center
New York, New York

Maus W. Stearns, Jr., M.D.
Former Chief, Rectum and Colon Service
Memorial Sloan-Kettering Cancer Center
New York, New York

Stephen S. Sternberg, M.D.
Attending Pathologist
Department of Pathology
Memorial Hospital
New York, New York

Harold J. Wanebo, M.D.
Chief, Division of Oncology
Department of Surgery
University of Virginia Medical Center
Charlottesville, Virginia

Horace W. Whiteley, Jr., M.D.
Associate Attending Surgeon
Rectum and Colon Service
Memorial Hospital
New York, New York

Sidney J. Winawer, M.D.
Chief, Gastroenterology Service
Memorial Sloan-Kettering Cancer Center
New York, New York

Preface

The intent of this monograph is to present the concepts of clinical management of patients with neoplasms of the colon, rectum, and anus that are shared by the Attending Staff of the Memorial Sloan-Kettering Cancer Center. These concepts, gathered from many sources, have been tempered by the combined experience of the staff. The marjority of these ideas were developed under the late Dr. George Binkley, who organized the Rectal and Colon Service at Memorial Hospital, and his successor, Dr. Michael Deddish. The validity of these concepts has stood the test of time and their application has been followed by results as satisfactory as any reported. It is our belief that future advances in management of these neoplasms will be made by additions to these basic principles, and that until more effective methods of management have been proved, these should remain the baseline.

Maus W. Stearns, Jr.

Contents

Neoplasms
of the Colon, Rectum,
and Anus

1
Epidemiology and Pathogenesis of Colorectal Cancer

Paul Sherlock

The etiology of cancer of the colon is not well understood, although in recent years substantial clues have been emerging. Although there are well-defined genetic syndromes that predispose to the development of colon cancer, environmental factors are believed to have the most significant role in the pathogenesis of colon neoplasia. Increased interest in nutrition and carcinogenesis has led to intensive clinical and laboratory investigation to define the possible roles of dietary factors in the pathogenesis of colon cancer.

Although the mechanism(s) whereby environmental factors interact with genetic and constitutional characteristics to predispose to colon cancer are largely unknown, certain alterations occur during the transformation of colon cells to the neoplastic state. It is the purpose of this review to outline the environmental, genetic, and cellular aspects that predispose to the development of carcinoma of the colon.

EPIDEMIOLOGY AND CARCINOGENESIS

The incidence of colon cancer is high in North America, northern and western Europe, and New Zealand and low in South America, Africa, and Asia. The United States has one of the highest rates of colon cancer in the world. With the exception of Japan, the disease is more prevalent in the developed countries, suggesting a relationship to economic development (1–3). Support for the concept that environmental factors are the most important is seen in the change in incidence in populations that migrate to an area where the incidence is different. This is well illustrated by the differing incidence of the disease among blacks living in America and those in Africa, Puerto Ricans living in Puerto Rico and those who have migrated to the mainland, and by the higher incidence of cancer of the colon in first- and second-generation Japanese immigrants to Hawaii and the mainland United States than in the Japanese in Japan. In the United States, statistics have shown that the incidence of colon cancer has been greater in the north than in the south; greater in urban areas than in rural areas; greater among Jewish than among non-Jewish people; and among white greater than among black people.

1

However, these patterns are changing, due largely to migrational shifts into urban areas, particularly evident in the white-black differences. It appears that immigrants to a particular geographic area assume the colon cancer risk of that area.

There is positive correlation between the incidence of colon cancer and economic development, general nutritional pattern, fat and protein consumption, and arteriosclerotic heart disease. There is no relationship to specific occupation except for a report of a higher incidence in asbestos workers (4), raising the speculation that chronic exposure to asbestos at low levels or exposure to other inorganic substances in the environment may be carcinogenic or promote carcinogenesis.

A substantial body of information and observations relates diet to the development of colon cancer. There is a low incidence of appendicitis, adenomatous polyps, diverticulosis, ulcerative colitis, and colon cancer in the South African Bantu and other African populations whose diets contain more fiber and roughage and less refined carbohydrates than is the case with diets in more developed areas (2). Their diets produce rapid intestinal transit, so that any potential carcinogen would be in contact with the mucosa for a shorter period of time.

Many investigators have suggested a direct association between increased fat and animal protein intake in the Western diet and the rising incidence of colon cancer. Beef intake may be the important factor contributing to the increasing incidence of colon cancer in New Zealand and Argentina. In Japan the intake of fat provides only 12% of the total caloric intake and is mostly of the unsaturated type, while in the United States fat intake represents 40 to 44% of the total caloric intake (5).

If diet determines the composition of microbial flora that may produce carcinogenic or cocarcinogenic compounds from food or gastrointestinal secretions, then dietary differences may explain the variation in geographic distribution of colon cancer. Greater population densities of anaerobic clostridia and bacteroides with fewer lactobacilli have been noted in populations at high risk for colon cancer. These are the only two organisms known to dehydrogenate the steroid nucleus—an effect that would be important for the development of compounds with structures similar to those of known carcinogens (6). It has been suggested that the Western diet, with its high beef and fat content, favors the establishment of a bacterial flora capable of producing enzymes such as beta glucuronidase and azoreductase with increased metabolic potential to metabolize acid and neutral sterols to carcinogens or cocarcinogens in the colon (7). In the experimental animal, rats fed either 20% lard or 20% corn oil were more susceptible to dimethylhydrazine-induced tumors than animals fed 5% lard or 5% corn oil (8). In animals, bile acids have been demonstrated to be promotors of 1,2-dimethylhydrazine (DMH)–induced and N-methyl-N′-nitrosoguanidine (MNNG)–induced cancers (9).

Inhibition of carcinogenesis may occur in natural and experimental situations. The microsomal enzyme, benzpyrene hydroxylase, located in the small intestine, protects against the carcinogenic effect of the polycyclic hydrocarbon benzpyrene. Foods that induce increased activity of benzpyrene hydroxylase include brussels sprouts, cabbage, turnips, broccoli, and cauliflower. This observation suggests that substances in the diet may protect against carcinogenesis by inducing cellular enzyme activity that detoxifies the luminal carcinogen (10). Also, certain phenolic antioxidants such as butylated hydroxyanesole (BHA) and butylated hydroxytoluene (BHT), which are added to foods to prevent oxidation, produce inhibition of experimental carcinogenesis (11).

Other antioxidants have been suggested as inhibitors of the neoplastic process. High selenium levels in the soil and foliage have been correlated with the low incidence of colon cancer in certain geographic areas in this country (12). Selenium fed to animals protects against the induction of cancer by dimethylhydrazine (13). Vitamin C (ascorbic acid) and vitamin E (alpha-tocopherol) have known antitumor effects in experimental animals, presumably from their antioxidant protection (14). In a preliminary study, administration of ascorbic acid to a group of patients with polyposis coli was associated with a reduction in the number and size of rectal adenomas (15).

The experimental use of vitamin A derivatives (retinoids) (16), as well as lactobacillus (7), has been associated with the inhibition of experimentally induced tumors. Various components of dietary fiber, such as lignin and pectin, can bind bile salts and their metabolites and increase their excretion, which may account for the apparent protective effect of fiber in colon carcinogenesis. Another possibility is that fiber, by increasing bulk, may dilute the potential carcinogen (2).

It is hoped that recent observations by Ames and others, using the *Salmonella typhimurium* mutagenesis assay, may identify those components in the diet that are mutagenic to the bacteria and therefore possibly carcinogenic to humans (17). Studies are under way in a number of laboratories attempting to define mutagenic activity in the feces. Bruce has demonstrated a mutagen nitrosamide in the feces of individuals on a meat diet. Reduction in mutagenicity and levels of nitrosamide in the stool has been noted in patients on high doses of ascorbic acid and alpha-tocopherol (18). The carcinogenic process is complex, with promoting and inhibiting factors interacting in unknown ways. Identification of these factors would certainly help define the carcinogenic process.

CELLULAR AND MOLECULAR CHANGES

The mode of interaction of carcinogens with colon cells has not been well defined. Hereditary processes in certain individuals undoubtedly influence and accelerate the development of colon neoplasia. During the neoplastic transformation of colon cells in humans and in experimental animals, proliferative abnormalities occur. The cells fail to repress DNA synthesis and to undergo normal differentiation, resulting in enhanced ability to proliferate. Maturing cells normally cease DNA synthesis and proliferative activity before they reach the surface of the mucosa. In humans, normal cells migrate to the surface of the mucosa in four to eight days and are extruded from the surface, and the entire lining of the colon mucosa is replaced with new cells. However, in patients with familial polyposis and other premalignant disorders, the epithelial cells, in patches of flat colon mucosa, begin to develop enhanced ability to synthesize DNA and to proliferate. This has been observed in morphologically normal-appearing colon epithelial cells in patients with familial polyposis before they develop adenomatous changes and before the cells begin to form polyps. It has been noted in 85% of random biopsy specimens (19).

In other areas of the colon, mucosa cells with persistent DNA synthesis develop additional properties enabling them to be retained in the mucosa in increasing numbers and to develop morphologic characteristics identified as adenomatous. As these excrescences enlarge and develop villous components, carcinomas develop with increasing frequency (20).

The development of neoplasia is associated with an increase in certain enzyme levels in colon cells that enable them to synthesize DNA and to proliferate. One such enzyme is thymidine-kinase, which is high in immature and low in well-differentiated colon cells

(21). The selective accumulation of certain nuclear proteins in colon cancer cells and the development of analytical procedures for their detection in single cells has been demonstrated (22). These newer observations offer a potential new approach to the early detection of molecular events in the development of malignancy prior to identifiable morphologic changes.

The identification of abnormal constituents in fecal contents, such as undegraded cholesterol, in patients with familial polyposis (23); the detection of well-defined immunologic abnormalities in families with a predisposition to colon cancer (24); and the behavior of skin fibroblasts in tissue culture from patients with familial polyposis (25) offer new approaches to the identification of individuals who may have increased susceptibility for the development of colon cancer.

GENETIC ASPECTS

Although current information suggests that most cancers involving the colon may have been influenced by environmental factors, in some instances genetic susceptibility may be the significant factor. The risk of cancer of the colon in relatives of patients with colorectal cancer is about three times that expected in the general population. There is suggestive evidence that patients under age 40 who develop colorectal carcinoma are more likely to have a family history of colorectal cancer than those over 40 who develop this cancer (5).

There are several well-defined genetic syndromes that predispose to the development of colorectal cancer. Familial polyposis is one such disorder, in which the population frequency has been estimated to be about 1 in 8,000 (26). An autosomal dominant mode of inheritance with a penetrance rate of 80% has been well established. It is estimated that two-thirds of patients with polyposis who present with symptoms will show evidence of cancer when first seen, and 50% will develop carcinoma by age 30. The mean age when diagnosis of cancer is made is about 40 years, 20 years sooner than colon cancer in the general population. Multiple cancers of the colon are commonly encountered. The duration of the polyposis phase averages about 10 years but may be as little as 5 years. Generally the polyps do not occur before puberty or initially after age 45 (27). Deschner and Lipkin, using short-term tissue-culture techniques to allow for isotope incorporation and incubating fragments of rectal mucosa and colon washings with tritiated thymidine, have demonstrated an extension of active DNA synthesis from the colon crypt cells to the surface cells (28).

Gardner's syndrome is another autosomal dominant disorder, with a frequency of 1 in 14,000. It is also characterized by adenomatous polyps of the colon. Sebaceous cysts, desmoid tumors, fibromas, epidermoid cysts, and osteomas may be present singly or in combination. Other associated conditions are abnormal dentition; thyroid, Ampulla of Vater, duodenal, and adrenal carcinomas; and carcinoid tumors. The Turcot syndrome, consisting of polyps of the colon in association with tumors of the central nervous system, and the Oldfield syndrome, with familial extensive sebaceous cysts, polyps of the colon, and adenocarcinoma, may merely be variants of Gardner's syndrome (27). The Peutz-Jeghers syndrome, with melanin pigmentation of the buccal mucosa, lips, face, fingers, anus, and vagina, is associated with hamartomatous polyps of the gastrointestinal tract, with little malignant potential. However, there have been some reports of associated carcinoma in the stomach, duodenum, and colon (29).

There are families whose members show a strikingly high incidence of malignancy at multiple sites, frequently in the endometrium and colon. These "cancer families" are characterized by early age of onset of the malignancies. Hereditary adenocarcinomatosis is the name of this disease entity, which is believed to be inherited as an autosomal dominant with 90% penetrance (30).

Juvenile polyposis of the colon is another inherited disorder, in which the polyps are actually hamartomas and are not considered premalignant. However, relatives of these patients do have an increased occurrence of both adenomatous polyps of the colon and colorectal carcinoma (30).

Cancer patients who have had partial resection of the colon are at increased risk for developing a new primary cancer in the remaining portion of the colon. In one series, a three-fold increase was noted. It is not clear whether genetic factors play a role here (31).

Adenomatous polyps occur in 5 to 10% of the general population. One or more polyps of the colon or rectum may be associated with the later development of adenocarcinoma. Kindreds have also been reported showing an association of single and multiple polyps and adenocarcinomas, an association that may be genetically determined. One reported kindred noted that 45% of the adult members of one generation had solitary polyps as well as polyps in multiple generations; there was a high incidence of adenocarcinomas of the colon in the family (32).

INFLAMMATORY BOWEL DISEASE

With ulcerative colitis, the likelihood of developing carcinoma at a later date is 3 to 5% (33), except in a recent study from continental Europe, in which no increase was noted (34). If this is compared to the prevalence of cancer of the colon and rectum in the general population, the risk of malignant change is 5 to 10 times greater. The risk is minimal prior to 10-years' duration of the colitis but begins to rise after 10 years, show-ing a more precipitous rise after 20 years. If ulcerative colitis develops before age 25, the risk of developing cancer may be double, compared to its development after age 25 (35). Other factors that increase the risk are total colon involvement, a clinically severe first attack, and chronic continuous symptoms, although relative freedom from symptoms does not indicate that a cancer will not develop.

In patients where cancer is superimposed on ulcerative colitis the malignancy usually occurs at least a decade earlier than in the general population. The cancer is more evenly distributed throughout the colon. A substantial number of tumors involve the transverse and ascending colon. The cancer can be multiple, it is frequently colloid and infiltrating, and it has a higher grade of malignancy than that occurring in the general population (33).

Granulomatous colitis had not previously been considered a premalignant disorder, but recently more cases associated with carcinoma have been reported with Crohn's disease of both the small and large bowel (36). In a recent study it was demonstrated that patients with Crohn's disease of the large bowel have 20 times the risk of develop-ing superimposed carcinoma of the large bowel (37). Most of the cancers were on the right side of the colon and most patients were under 40 years of age. Clinicians can no longer dismiss the possibility of a cancer risk in patients with this disease. Vigorous sur-veillance is needed.

POLYPS

There is a substantial body of information that favors the concept that adenomatous polyps are precursors of colon cancer (27). About one-third of all specimens from operations for colorectal cancer have one or more adenomatous polyps (38). There are many documented examples of invasive carcinoma in continuity with recognizable adenomatous tissue, with a spectrum of change from benign adenomatous tissue to dysplasia or atypia, to focal cancer, to invasive cancer. The peak incidence of adenomatous polyps occurs about 5 to 10 years sooner than the peak incidence of colorectal carcinoma with merely a shift to the left in the age distribution curve. Cellular atypia becomes increasingly more evident as the polyp increases in size, with abnormal chromosome patterns increasing with the greater degree of atypia. Experimental carcinogens produce both polyps and cancer in animal models (39). In familial polyposis the many adenomatous polyps have a histologic appearance similar to that of adenomas observed elsewhere, and cancer develops from the polyp rather than in the flat mucosa between the polypoid lesions. Early cancer with minute mucosal lesions has not been seen, which is to be expected if colorectal cancer arises de novo from flat mucosa (40). Finally, in Gilbertsen's study, removing all polyps from the rectosigmoid on annual sigmoidoscopic examination lessened the incidence of cancer of the rectosigmoid as compared to a retrospective control population (41).

There are arguments against the concept that adenomatous polyps are precursors of colorectal cancer (42), but the available evidence suggests the premalignant nature of some polyps. Only about 5% of polyps become malignant, and it takes at least 5 years for them to do so. The important questions are: Why do most polyps not become malignant? How can one predict those that will eventually develop malignant transformation?

CONCLUSIONS

Most colon cancers may ultimately be determined to have been caused by one or more environmental factors. It would appear from epidemiologic studies, particularly migrant studies, that colorectal carcinoma is related to a more affluent and industrialized civilization and change of life style. Diets rich in fat may alter the bacterial flora, which in turn may produce carinogens or cocarcinogens from the gastrointestinal secretory metabolites. Inhibition of carcinogenesis by antioxidants and fiber may play a modifying role. Change at the cellular level includes an enhanced ability for cellular DNA synthesis and proliferation, and a change in surface enzymes.

Experiments with animal models have added to the information obtained in humans as to the specific changes that occur during the neoplastic transformation of colon cells. Modification by genetic and immunologic factors undoubtedly occur and there are specific syndromes in which the genetic aspects seem paramount. Chronic, long-standing inflammation, as in ulcerative colitis and granulomatous colitis, also predisposes to the development of cancer of the colon. The premalignant nature of adenomatous polyps remains a subject of controversy, but the existing evidence favors a relationship, although only a small number of polyps develop malignant change. Further studies are needed to clarify the exact role of diet and environmental factors in the development of colorectal cancer.

REFERENCES

1. Wynder EL: The epidemiology of large bowel cancer. *Cancer Res* 35:3388, 1975.

2. Walker ARP, Burkitt DP: Colon cancer: Epidemiology. *Seminars in Oncol* 3:341, 1976.

3. Weisburger JH, Reddy BS, Wynder EL: Colon cancer: Its epidemiology and experimental production. *Cancer* 40:2414, 1977.

4. Selikoff IJ, Churg J, Hammond EC: Asbestos exposure and neoplasia. *JAMA* 188:22, 1964.

5. Wynder EL, Shigematsu T: Environmental factors of cancer of the colon and rectum. *Cancer* 20:1520, 1967.

6. Hill MJ: The role of colon anaerobes in the metabolism of bile acids and steroids and its relation to colon cancer. *Cancer* 36:2387, 1975.

7. Goldin BR, Gorbach SL: The relationship between diet and rat fecal bacterial enzymes implicated in colon cancer. *J Natl Cancer Inst* 57:371, 1976.

8. Reddy BS, Narisawa T, Maronput R, et al: Animal models for the study of dietary factors and cancer of the large bowel. *Cancer Res* 35:3421, 1975.

9. Narisawa T, Magadia NE, Weisburger JH, Wynder EL: Promoting effect of bile acid on colon carcinogenesis after intrarectal instillation of N-methyl-N'-nitrosoguanidine in rats. *J Natl Cancer Inst* 55:1093, 1974.

10. Wattenberg LW: Studies of polycyclic hydrocarbon hydroxylases of the intestine possibly related to cancer. Effect of diet on benzpyrene hydroxylase activity. *Cancer* 26:99, 1971.

11. Wattenberg LW: Potential inhibitors of colon carcinogenesis. *Am J Digest Dis* 19:947, 1974.

12. Shamberger RJ, Rukovena E, Longfeld AR, et al: Antioxidants and cancer. I. Selenium in the blood of normal and cancer patients. *J Natl Cancer Inst* 50:863, 1973.

13. Jacobs MM: Inhibitory effect of selenium on 1,2-dimethylhydrazine and methylazoxymethanol colon carcinogenesis: Correlative studies on the mutagenecity and sister chromatid exchange rates of selected carcinogens. *Cancer* 40:2557, 1977.

14. Pamukcu AM, Valciner S, Bryan GT: Inhibition of carcinogenic effect of brachen fern (Pteridium aquilinum) by various chemicals. *Cancer* 40:2450, 1977.

15. DeCosse JJ, Adams MG, Kuzma JF, LoGerfo P, Condon RE: Effect of ascorbic acid on rectal polyps of patients with familial polyposis. *Surgery* 78:608, 1975.

16. Sporn MB, Dunlop NM, Newton DL, Smith JM: Prevention of chemical carcinogenesis by vitamin A and its synthetic analogs (retinoids). *Fed Proc* 35:1332, 1976.

17. Ames BN, McCann J, Yamasaki E: Methods for detecting carcinogens and mutagens with the Salmonella/mammalian microsome mutagenecity test. *Mutat Res* 31:347, 1975.

18. Bruce WR: Discussion at the American Gastroenterological Association Symposium on The Environment and Gastrointestinal Cancer. Las Vegas, May 1978.

19. Deschner EE, Lipkin M: Study of human rectal epithelial cells *in vitro* III. RNA protein and DNA synthesis in polyps and adjacent mucosa. *J Natl Cancer Inst* 44:175, 1970.

20. Lipkin M: Phase I and phase II proliferative lesions of colonic epithelial cells in diseases leading to colonic cancer. *Cancer* 34:878, 1974.

21. Salser JS, Balis ME: Distribution and regulation of deoxythymidine kinase activity in differentiating cells of mammalian intestines. *Cancer Res* 33:1889, 1973.

22. Boffa LC, Allfrey VG: Characteristic complements of nuclear non-histone proteins in colonic epithelial tumors. *Cancer Res* 36:2678, 1976.

23. Reddy BS, Mastromarino A, Gustafson C, et al: Fecal bile acids and neutral sterols in patients with familial polyposis. *Cancer* 38:1694, 1976.

24. Berlinger NT, Lopez C, Lipkin M, et al: Defective recognitive immunity on family aggregates of colon cancer. *J Clin Invest* 59:761, 1977.

25. Pfeffer LM, Kopelovich L: Differential genetic susceptibility of cultured human skin fibroblasts to transformation by Kirsten Murine Sarcoma Virus. *Cell* 10:313, 1977.

26. Reed TE, Heel JW: A genetic study of multiple polyposis of the colon. *Am J Human Genetics* 7:236, 1955.

27. Sherlock P, Lipkin M, Winawer SJ: Predisposing factors in carcinoma of the colon. *Advances Int Med* 20:121, 1975.

28. Deschner EE, Lewis CM, Lipkin M. *In vitro* study of human epithelial cells. I. Atypical zone of H³ thymidine incorporation in mucosa of multiple polyposis. *J Clin Invest* 42:1922, 1963.

29. Dodds WJ, Schalle WJ, Henley GT, Hogan WJ: Peutz-Jegher's syndrome and gastrointestinal malignancy. *Am J Roentgenol* 115:374, 1972.

30. Lynch HT, Krush AJ: Heredity and adenocarcinoma of the colon. *Gastroenterology* 53:517, 1967.

31. Schottenfeld D, Berg JW, Vitsky B: Incidence of multiple primary cancers. *J Natl Cancer Inst* 43:77, 1969.

32. Woolf CM, Richards RC, Gardner EJ: Occasional discrete polyps of colon and rectum showing inherited tendency in kindred. *Cancer* 8:403, 1955.

33. Morson BC: Cancer in ulcerative colitis. *Gut* 7:425, 1966.

34. Binder V, Bonnevic O, Gertz T, et al: Ulcerative colitis in children: Treatment cause and prognosis. *Scand J Gastroenterol* 8:161, 1973.

35. MacDougall IPM: The cancer risk in ulcerative colitis. *Lancet* 2:655, 1964.

36. Lightdale CJ, Sternberg SS, Posner G, Sherlock P: Carcinoma complicating Crohn's disease. *Am J Med* 59:262, 1975.

37. Weedon DD, Shorter RG, Ilstrup DM, et al: Crohn's disease and cancer. *N Engl J Med* 289:1099, 1973.

38. Morson BC, Bussey H Jr: Predisposing causes of intestinal cancer, in Ravitch M (ed): *Current Problems in Surgery*. Chicago, Year Book Medical Publishers, Inc, 1970.

39. Thurnherr N, Deschner EE, Stonehill EH, Lipkin M: Induction of adenocarcinoma of the colon in mice by weekly injections of 1,2-dimethylhydrazine. *Cancer Res* 33:940, 1973.

40. Stearns MW: Where are the tiny carcinomas of the rectum? *Surg Gynecol Obstet* 116:625, 1963.

41. Gilbertsen VA: Proctosigmoidoscopy and polypectomy in reducing the incidence of rectal cancer. *Cancer* 34:936, 1974.

42. Castleman B, et al: Carcinoma arising in adenomatous polyps of the colon is greatly exaggerated, in Ingelfinger FJ, Rebman AA, Finland M (eds): *Controversy in Internal Medicine*. Philadelphia, WB Saunders Co, 1966.

2
Early Diagnosis of Colorectal Cancer

Sidney J. Winawer

SYMPTOMATIC PATIENTS

Most patients with colorectal cancer seek medical attention after symptoms have occurred. However, if patients delay seeking medical attention for some time after the onset of symptoms, personal morbidity and the risk of mortality are greatly increased. Further delay by the physician who first sees the patient with such symptoms may be critical (1).

Comparative studies for other cancers agree with this observation; less delay in diagnosing and treating breast cancer, for example, is correlated with smaller lesions and better survival (2). Whereas the presence of symptoms in patients with colorectal cancer is related to a less favorable prognosis, these symptoms may be associated with a premalignant lesion such as an adenoma or ulcerative colitis rather than a cancer. The importance of a thorough investigation of symptomatic patients is, therefore, related not only to a diagnosis of colorectal cancer but also to a possible premalignant disease, which, if treated properly, could have an important impact on the patients' future risk for colorectal cancer. For this reason, symptomatic patients, especially those with rectal bleeding, must be studied aggressively with roentgenography and endoscopy. This approach will, of course, be modified by the risk factors present; for example, a 21-year-old woman with rectal bleeding and no other associated risk factor may be worked up less aggressively than a 21-year-old woman with a strong family history of colon cancer or a 50-year-old woman, regardless of the presence or absence of associated risk factors (Table 1). Symptoms that require investigation include: rectal bleeding; a recent change in the caliber of stools to a thinner stool; a recent change in bowel habits, with recent onset of either constipation or diarrhea; and constipation, indicating the possibility of a left colon lesion, or diarrhea, indicating the possibility of a lesion anywhere in the colon, but especially on the right side. There are other symptoms that are associated with benign disorders of the colon that also suggest the possibility of malignancy and require investigation, such as increased mucous discharge from the rectum as a possible indication of a villous adenoma and the onset of new symptoms of vague abdominal pain, increased flatus, and "irritable bowel syndrome," all of which could signal the presence of early, partially obstructing, colon cancer. These symptoms may be especially disturbing when they are new symptoms in adults who have not had long-standing symptoms of functional bowel disease. We now have available all the methods necessary for adequate clarification of the underlying nature of these symptoms (3).

Table 1. Colorectal Cancer Risk Factors

Standard Risk	Age over 40, men and women
High Risk	Inflammatory bowel disease
	History of female genital or breast cancer
	History of colon cancer or adenoma
	Peutz-Jegher's syndrome
	Familial polyposis syndromes
	Family cancer syndromes
	Hereditary site-specific colon cancer
	History of juvenile polyps
	Immunodeficiency disease

Diagnostic Methods

Sigmoidoscopy

A digital rectal examination and sigmoidoscopy should be the first step in the diagnostic evaluation of patients with symptoms suggestive of neoplasia. Digital examination is of critical importance since posterior lesions above the sphincter may be missed on endoscopy. Approximately 50% of invasive carcinomas of the colon and rectum will be detectable within range of an adequate sigmoidoscopy. However, the maximum value of this procedure is often not obtained by the inexperienced examiner, who may not consistently insert the sigmoidoscope beyond 17 or 18 cm. In addition, it has been shown that, unless the bowel is telescoped and the proper insertion procedure is followed, the bowel may be stretched to 25 cm, although only 17 or 18 cm of mucosa is examined. Very few examiners compress and look behind each rectal valve to search for hidden lesions. The value of this procedure increases with the experience of the examiner. It is particularly important to perform a sigmoidoscopy before a barium enema. The barium enema fails to reveal a significant number of rectal lesions. In addition, the patient's symptoms may be caused by a low-lying lesion in the rectosigmoid that is partially obstructing and could result in a perforation during the barium enema if the radiologist is not alerted to such a lesion.

The patient's symptoms of rectal bleeding could be due to benign disease such as inflammatory bowel disease with a friable mucosa, which would contraindicate a barium enema until adequate treatment resulted in improvement of mucosal friability. In addition to cancer, a significant percentage of adenomas are detectable by this method. New instrumentation is being developed in sigmoidoscopy with application of fiber optics to this technique. Several flexible sigmoidoscopes are currently available. The 60-cm length of these instruments provides the potential for a more comprehensive examination of the distal bowel but requires greater expertise of the examiner. The higher yield of the flexible technique at present is offset by not only the necessary expertise required but the higher cost of purchase and maintenance of the instruments. These instruments are undergoing preliminary trials at the present time and their true value must await further evaluation (4,5).

Air-Contrast Barium Enema

This method is exceedingly important in the orderly investigation of the symptomatic patient. The barium enema when properly performed will complement sigmoidoscopy and will also complement colonoscopy. The area where the barium enema complements colonoscopy best is the right side of the colon in patients in whom colonoscopy has not reached the right side or in whom the examination of the right side is suboptimal. Experienced endoscopists can reach the cecum in approximately 90% of patients examined. Other areas that are potentially blind during colonoscopy, and for which a good barium enema is a complementary procedure, are the hepatic and splenic flexures. A mass detected on a barium enema will also alert the endoscopist to an area of interest. A low-lying left colon cancer, especially a partially obstructing cancer of the sigmoid, may obviate the need for further endoscopic examination. In addition, in some patients a normal sigmoidoscopy together with a normal barium enema may eliminate the need for further diagnostic studies if symptoms are marginal. For example, patients with long-standing irritable bowel syndrome who may present to a physician for the first time and are at standard risk for colorectal cancer only by virtue of being over 40 years old, in whom the physician may wish to proceed with a reasonable diagnostic investigation but not an overly aggressive one, may have the workup ended if the sigmoidoscopy and barium enema are both perfectly normal. Unfortunately, the barium enema is often suboptimal because of poor preparation by the patient or because of the omission of the air-contrast technique. The regular barium enema without good air contrast can miss as much as 40% of the polypoid lesions and 20% of carcinomas as compared to a good air-contrast barium enema (Table 2) (6). Malmo-type air-contrast barium enema techniques can detect the majority of polyps >1 cm in size but will still miss many of the lesions <1 cm (7).

Colonoscopy

This technique has revolutionized our diagnostic capabilities in dealing with colonic disease and will become even more important in the investigation of patients suspected of having colorectal neoplasia. Polyps and cancer not detected by barium enema have been detected frequently by colonoscopy (7,8). Patients should be considered for colonoscopy who present with symptoms suggesting neoplastic disease, especially occult or gross bleeding, and have a negative barium enema; to clarify an equivocal barium enema; to confirm a positive barium enema; and to search for additional sychronous lesions (9). A previous study, in which colotomy and intraoperative rigid endoscopy were used, demonstrated additional adenomas in 47% of 103 patients in whom the diagnosis of colonic polyps had been made. Forty percent of these additional adenomas were >1 cm in diameter and carcinoma was found in approximately 25% of all patients with a preoperative diagnosis of a benign polyp, often at a second site (10). Not everyone agrees that the patient with a lesion seen on barium enema that is convincing for a colon cancer needs preoperative colonoscopy for confirmation of that diagnosis. However, it is becoming increasingly accepted in the medical community that a patient having one

Table 2. Comparison of Barium Enema with Air Contrast and Colonoscopy in Detection of Polyps

	Barium Enema	Colonoscopy
Polyps > 5 mm	21	37
Polyps < 5 mm	3	30
	24	67

Table 3. Diagnosis of Cancer by Colonoscopic Biopsy and Cytology: Influence of Growth Pattern on Accuracy of Tissue Diagnosis

	Number Positive			
Technique	Infiltrative Cancer		Exophytic Cancer	
Biopsy	4/12	(33%)	20/28	(71%)
Biopsy and lavage	4/9	(44%)	15/16	(94%)
Biopsy and brush	7/9	(78%)	17/18	(94%)
Biopsy, brush, and lavage	5/6	(83%)	12/13	(92%)

Reprinted with permission of the publishers of *Cancer* 42:2849–2853, 1978.

colorectal neoplasm stands a 40 to 50% chance of having a second synchronous adenoma (11), and a 3 to 5% chance of having a second synchronous colon cancer (12).

It is not sufficient, therefore, to operate on a patient for a lesion demonstrated on x-ray film without clearing the colon of additional lesions. The endoscopy can either be done at the time of surgery by intraoperative rigid endoscopy or at some time perioperatively, by colonoscopy. Preoperative colonoscopy can clear the colon distal to the neoplastic lesion. This approach can have a major beneficial effect on right colon and transverse colon lesions. In the presence of left colon lesions, especially those in the sigmoid, the problem is a more difficult one. Although we would wish to clear the entire remaining colon of synchronous lesions, many endoscopists do not feel comfortable passing through a segment of colon with a known carcinoma, especially if it is a partially obstructing one. The method and timing of this approach can be individualized to the particular patient, but the concept is a valid one that at some time, perioperatively, additional lesions must be carefully searched for.

Biopsy and Cytology

When specific lesions are seen, target biopsy and target brush cytology have a high diagnostic yield (Table 3) (13). Biopsy can be done through any of the rigid or flexible sigmoidoscopes, and biopsy and brush cytology can be performed through any of the flexible instruments. The value and the yield of the cytological approach requires a good cytological laboratory and an interested gastrointestinal cytologist. Lavage cytology has to a large extent been replaced by direct target techniques and is now reserved for select situations, such as the surveillance of high-risk groups (Table 1). Lavage through a flexible scope may also be helpful when there is a mass lesion in a fixed bowel, the nature of which is unclear, and the lesion cannot be reached by the scope. An example of this is the patient with diverticular disease and a mass lesion that appear on x-ray film. Gentle lavage, using saline, through the flexible scope with aspiration of fluid into a trap filled with 95% alcohol can result in diagnosis of malignancy on smears from this fluid. If possible, however, it is preferable to use brush cytology rather than lavage, since brushing results in two or three smears with a high concentration of cells compared to the many more smears produced by lavage, each with a much lower concentration of cells and considerable debris. Brush cytology has also been useful in the clarification of the nature of strictures in inflammatory bowel disease. Thorough brushing from within the stricture is often productive of diagnostic cells.

The concept of false-positive cytology has been overly emphasized in the literature. We have rarely seen a false-positive cytology in the absence of malignancy. In the few cases that we have seen this, the patients have had severe underlying premalignant disease such as familial polyposis, or long-standing ulcerative colitis. The malignant-appearing cells under these circumstances may merely represent severely atypical cellular changes or could be the first indication of biological malignancy, manifest cytologically, without groups of tumor cells on histological section. On rare occasions a benign polyp without any histologic malignancy can result in a positive brushing or washing for malignant cells. Considering the frequency of malignant change in adenomas, the low incidence of false-positive cytology in these lesions is interesting.

ASYMPTOMATIC PATIENTS

Risk factors for colorectal cancer may be seen in Table 1. The age risk begins in men and women at age 40 and begins to rise more steeply at age 50, doubling with each subsequent decade (14). The age factor is modified by family history, those people who have a strong family history of colorectal cancer may begin to have increased risk at a younger age. Increased risk begins at age 21 for site-specific familial colon cancer and familial colon cancer associated with cancers at multiple anatomic sites, especially female genital cancer. These lesions are primarily on the right side (15). Patients in families with the familial polyposis syndromes usually begin to have an increased risk at puberty, the time at which affected individuals begin to manifest polyposis. The average age of diagnosis of the polyposis is 25, and the average age of diagnosis of cancer in this group is 40, which is considerably younger than the average age of colorectal cancer seen in the general population. Cancers are usually advanced in these patients if the diagnosis is made at the time they are symptomatic.

The polyposis syndromes are inherited as a Mendelian dominant with a high degree of penetrance (16). Familial polyposis results in carpeting of the colon with hundreds of small polyps. Gardner's syndrome is a variant of familial polyposis associated with a variety of soft tissue and bony tumors, including fibromas, desmoids, and osteomas. Some of these patients may also have polyps in the stomach. The latter seems to be more common in affected Japanese, and the extent to which gastric polyposis occurs in Americans with this disease is not clear. There are other rare variants of the familial polyposis syndromes, including Turcot's syndrome, which has associated tumors of the central nervous system (CNS) and Oldfields' syndrome, which has associated sebaceous cysts.

Juvenile polyposis was previously thought to be a benign disorder, and it is still considered to be benign for the individual at the time the diagnosis is made; however, the individual and the family appear to be at high risk for future development of colorectal adenomas and cancer. The Peutz-Jegher's syndrome, also previously thought to be a perfectly benign disorder, may be associated with a variety of gastrointestinal neoplasms, including colorectal adenomas and cancer. In a significant number of patients with multiple polyposis, no familial history can be obtained. Patients with sporadic neoplastic polyps are also at higher risk for colon cancer, especially those with villous adenomas or villous components in adenomatous polyps. The evidence that adenomas are premalignant include the following: about one-third of operative specimens for colon cancer have one or more adenomatous polyps; invasive cancer has been documented frequently in conjunction with adenomatous tissue; there is increasing cellular atypia with growth of the polyp; and in familial polyposis the multiple adenomatous polyps have a histological appearance similar to that of the adenomas observed in the individual polyp.

Although the polyp/cancer controversy has not yet been completely resolved and is comprehensively reviewed elsewhere (9), it may be wiser to consider patients with polyps to be at higher risk for colon cancer, particularly at present, with the availability of techniques for detection and removal. Patients who have had a previous colon cancer are also at higher risk for a second colon cancer, the metachronous rate for subsequent cancers being approximately 4%. The presence of adenomatous polyps in the resected specimen further increases the risk of future colon cancer six-fold.

Ulcerative colitis is frequently associated with later malignancy. The incidence of malignancy begins to rise after 7 years, with a sharper rise after 20 years, and has been reported to be as high as 20 to 30% in some series. Risk is higher with universal disease as compared to left-sided disease, and least or negligible with rectal involvement only. The average age of onset of the cancer is about 40, which is younger than the average age of onset of colon cancer in the general population, and the cancers tend to be multicentric and more uniformly distributed throughout the colon, as compared to the more left-sided distribution, generally. Granulomatous colitis is also considered premalignant but of a lower order of magnitude (17–20).

Screening Methods

Sigmoidoscopy

The value of this procedure in detecting colon cancer early in asymptomatic people has been well established in many centers. An estimate of the yield of invasive cancer on proctosigmoidoscopy in asymptomatic patients over the age of 40 is 1.5 in 1,000, or 1 in every 667 patients examined initially (21–24). In a study at the Preventive Medicine Institute-Strang Clinic, 58 cancers were detected in over 26,000 mostly asymptomatic patients during 47,000 examinations (21). Of the 50 patients followed for 15 or more years the survival was close to 90% (25), which is striking compared to the usual five-year survival of less than 50% for cancer of the colon.

The effort, cost, and acceptability of sigmoidoscopy limits its usefulness as a widely applied screening method for the general population. However, its value in the control of colon cancer cannot be related to the rate of detection of frank carcinoma alone. Adenomas are a much more common finding than cancer. The prevalence of polyps on proctosigmoidoscopy in patients over 40 years of age was reported to vary from 4 to 9% in several studies (21–24). Our own experience is more in the range of 2 to 4% for true adenomas at the first examination. The importance of adenoma detection is in the interruption of the polyp/cancer sequence by their removal. In one study, removal of rectosigmoid adenomas resulted in a lower than expected (15%) incidence of rectosigmoid cancer in a group of 18,000 patients followed for 25 years (26).

Sigmoidoscopy has not enjoyed popularity among physicians or patients in this country as a screening method in the asymptomatic patient. However, because of its effectiveness annual screening, which should not be equated with periodic screening, may not be required. A low risk for rectosigmoid cancer has been observed in people for three or four years after they have had one negative sigmoidoscopy (26). This is reasonable considering the gradual development of adenomas from normal mucosa and the long time they require to grow to significant size with premalignant potential. There may be, therefore, no advantage in having a sigmoidoscopy more often than every three to five years for screening purposes. The introduction of flexible sigmoidoscopy has been in part an attempt to increase patient and physician acceptance of this procedure and an attempt to increase the potential diagnostic yield of this approach, since the flexible instrument can examine an area that is beyond the reach of the rigid scope. In preliminary studies reported to date, flexible sigmoidoscopy has demonstrated a higher yield of neoplastic lesions as compared to rigid sigmoidoscopy (Table 4). Considerably more information will be required to evaluate the comparative yields of the two techniques.

Barium Enema

This method is too costly and time-consuming to be considered as a screening procedure in asymptomatic patients. It has obvious value in the orderly investigation of patients with symptoms. Although these statements are true in general for the population at standard risk by virtue of age, there may be some exceptions to the use of the barium enema as a screening test. For example, in patients with familial site-specific colon cancer there is a high risk of right-sided colon cancer. Under these circumstances the complementary use of a good air-contrast barium enema and colonoscopy on a periodic basis may be the only way to comfortably rule out the presence of right-sided colon cancer in these high-risk patients. Less invasive tests such as fecal occult blood tests can, of course, be used in these patients for interval screening but may not be sufficient when complete screening is called for. Barium enema and colonoscopy must also be used periodically in patients who have had a previously identified colon neoplasm, including adenoma and cancer. Under these circumstances also one cannot rely on fecal occult blood testing as a screening procedure because of the low sensitivity of the fecal occult blood test for new adenomas, which we would be searching for in these patients.

Colonoscopy

Colonoscopy complements the barium enema exceedingly well in the comprehensive workup of patients in any of the high-risk groups. Its value is in the detection of cancers not detected by barium enema, in the detection of adenomas missed by the barium enema, and in the detection of additional synchronous lesions. Followup surveillance in high-risk groups cannot be considered to be complete without the use of colonoscopy because of the above reasons.

Table 4. Comparison of Abnormalities Detected by Rigid and Flexible Sigmoidoscopy (108 Patients)[a]

	Rigid Sigmoidoscopy	Flexible Sigmoidoscopy
Cancer	1	5
Polyps > 5 mm	2	20
Polyps < 5 mm	1	15
Diverticulosis	1	13

[a] Reproduced with permission of the publishers of *Digestive Diseases and Sciences* 24:277–281, 1979.

Biopsy and Cytology

These techniques have considerable value in high-risk patients who are asymptomatic. Lesions detected in these patients can be assessed cytologically and histologically by these methods and, in certain high-risk groups, if no specific lesions are seen, lavage cytology can be done. Lavage cytology is routinely done during endoscopic surveillance examinations in patients with familial polyposis and in patients with long-standing inflammatory bowel disease. In patients with inflammatory bowel disease, the cancers may be flat and may not be visible by either colonoscopy or barium enema and may be detected by lavage cytology. Our approach is to do an annual colonoscopy with lavage in patients with inflammatory bowel disease of more than 7 years' duration who are not to undergo surgery. The same approach is used in patients with granulomatous colitis, who have a higher risk for malignancy than the general population but of a lower order of magnitude compared to patients with long-standing ulcerative colitis. In the followup endoscopic examination of patients having had a prior resection for colorectal cancer, the anastomosis is routinely brushed even though it may have a normal appearance. This technique can sometimes pick up a recurrence that is not apparent by either roentgenography or colonoscopy (Fig. 1).

Endoscopic biopsy can be of importance in assessing the extent of colonic involvement of ulcerative colitis and in assessing the premalignant potential of the mucosa. In

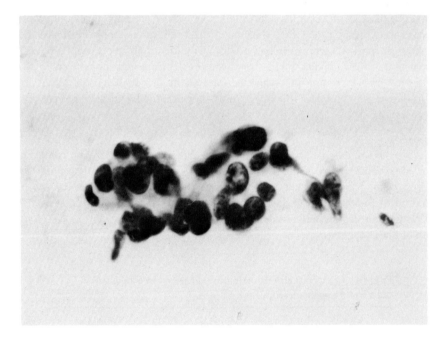

Figure 1. Malignant cells having large nuclei with coarsely granular chromatin, prominent nucleoli, and scanty cytoplasm. Cells were obtained by brush cytology from slightly irregular anastomosis in a man with previous colon cancer who now presented with Hemoccult-positive slides, normal x-ray films, and no symptoms. A small Dukes' A carcinoma was present at surgery. (Papanicolaou ×350). (Reprinted from *Seminars in Oncology* 3:387–392, 1976, with permission of the publishers, Grune & Stratton, New York).

patients with distal colitis determined by sigmoidoscopy but with normal barium enema and normal colonoscopy, colonoscopic biopsy of the more proximal colon may yield histological evidence of involvement that would then place the patient in the category of pancolitis, requiring greater surveillance for carcinoma, rather than in the lower-risk category of distal ulcerative colitis. The studies of Morson and associates suggest that biopsies in the rectosigmoid could indicate the presence of malignancy higher up in the colon (27). They have demonstrated that a small percentage of patients with long-standing ulcerative colitis show histological evidence of severe dysplasia, which is correlated with a high risk for malignancy. This approach requires multiple biopsies in a quiescent colon and interpretation by a pathologist with considerable experience in this concept. There are very few pathologists in this country at the present time who feel sufficiently comfortable with this concept to use it as part of the management of these patients. Biopsies obtained higher up by colonoscopy may indicate the presence of dysplasia not seen on rectal biopsies (27).

Biopsy and brush cytology are not generally used for evaluation of benign-appearing polyps. These lesions are only biopsied or brushed if a malignancy is suspected. The histological nature of benign-appearing polyps is best evaluated by total excision of the polyp by either snare cautery or by surgical removal. We usually remove benign-appearing pedunculated polyps by colonoscopic snare cautery technique regardless of size. We also remove most sessile lesions that appear benign and are under 2 cm in size. We do not attempt to remove malignant lesions, whether pedunculated or sessile, and we are reluctant to remove sessile lesions that exceed 2 cm in size since total excision of these lesions without subsequent recurrence is difficult. There is also a likelihood of malignancy in sessile lesions of 2 cm or more (28). Although removal of large sessile lesions by colonoscopy has been reported, there is little follow-up information regarding recurrence, incidence of carcinoma, need for additional surgery, and complication rate. Polyps 3 to 5 mm in size can be removed by hot biopsy, which is a combination of biopsy and fulguration. Excrescences of 1 to 3 mm in size are usually left alone since they are frequently seen and are usually hyperplasias.

Fecal Occult Blood Testing

There has been renewed interest in the test for occult blood in the stool. Testing of random stools on an unmodified diet has been shown to be worthless because of many false negatives and false positives. Guaiac solutions have had too many false positives. Hematest has been shown to be unreliable, and Benzidine too sensitive (29). The impregnated guaiac slide test (Smithkline Diagnostics, Sunnyvale, Calif) has been shown to be of value as a screening test for colonic neoplasia when used in a prescribed way; two slides prepared by the patient at home from different parts of the stool each day for three days for a total of six slides, while the patient is on a meat-free, high-roughage diet (30,31). This has been shown to detect blood, the investigation of which has led to the finding of early asymptomatic colon cancer in a number of studies (30–35).

False positives and false negatives can occur with this test. False positives occur since this test is based on the detection of blood and is not specific for neoplasia. Any bleeding lesion, therefore, can result in a positive test, including hemorrhoids, angiodysplasia, contamination by menstrual blood, and bleeding caused by aspirin-containing analgesics (Table 5). The peroxidase activity of some vegetables can also produce a false positive, since the color change of the guaiac is based on peroxidase. False negatives can occur when the patient is not on a high-bulk diet, which irritates potentially bleeding lesions;

Table 5. False-Positive Fecal Occult-Blood Testing

Noncompliance with diet
Aspirin compounds
Anticoagulants
Menstruation
Nonneoplastic bleeding lesions

when the patient does not smear the stools adequately; in the presence of vitamin C, which interferes with the reaction; or when the lesion is not bleeding at the time the stools are smeared (Table 6) (36). In addition, it has been shown that smears that have blood and are stored for several days may lose their reactivity because of desiccation (37–39). It has been shown that rehydration with a few drops of water prior to testing will restore this reactivity in such stools (40), but the restoration of reactivity with water may result in a reaction that is too sensitive, producing many false positives. The concept of rehydration is a valid one, but at the present time in our program we are not performing this because we suspect that it is producing too many false positives by an overly sensitive reaction resulting from this technique (41).

Apparently iron, laxatives, and barium do not interfere with this test, although it would be sensible not to have any of these used at the time the testing is done (38). Since this test is based on a commercial product, it depends on manufacturing control of the product and the sensitivity of the guaiac slide, which may change from time to time. For example, it appears that the Hemoccult II® slide currently in use is more sensitive than the single Hemoccult® slide previously used, but the former is not so sensitive that it produces many false positives (41). This increased sensitivity is thus beneficial in contrast to the rehydration sensitivity. The efficacy of the meat-free diet has been questioned by some, but the evidence in the literature suggests that for the present time such a diet should be used. Although its importance is not completely established, it seems reasonable not to increase the possibility of false positives by the use of meat in the diet, which may result in increased peroxidase activity in the stool from myoglobin and animal blood.

The use of the Hemoccult slide to date suggests that it has potential usefulness in the approach to screening in asymptomatic patients. It is obviously of no value in patients with underlying bleeding disease such as ulcerative colitis and familial polyposis. It should also not be the only screening test used in patients who have already been identified as high risk for colorectal neoplasms by virtue of other risk factors (see Table 1). In the initial series by Greegor, 5% of the patients had positive tests (30,31), but he has indicated that, in his recent personal experience, about 1% of his patients had posi-

Table 6. False-Negative Fecal Occult-Blood Testing

Noncompliance with diet
Noncompliance with slides
Nonbleeding of neoplasia
Sampling error
Vitamin C
Storage of prepared slides

tive tests (42). The cancers detected in his experience were primarily early cancers without lymph node involvement and without metastases. In a collaborative study in which 103 physicians reported on the use of this approach, 139 cancers were detected, with one patient having a false-negative test. In 47 resected cases that were considered to be truly silent, without symptoms and without anemia, 85% were localized pathologically, compared to the national average of 42% of detected colon cancers being localized. Only 20 of these cancers were within reach of the rigid sigmoidoscope (30,31). Other studies noted above support the favorable results of Greegor's initial observation.

There are two controlled trials of fecal occult blood testing under way at the present time, one at Memorial Sloan-Kettering Cancer Center in collaboration with the Preventive Medicine Institute-Strang Clinic and one at the University of Minnesota. In both these studies, the rate of positive slides initially was 1 to 2% (11,43). In our series, approximately 50% of the patients with positive slides had significant neoplastic lesions, including cancers, 12%, and adenomas, 38%. The remaining 50% of the patients with positive slides had nonneoplastic lesions. The University of Minnesota experience paralleled these results fairly closely. With current use of the new Hemoccult II slide test it appears that the rate of positive slides has increased to 3.5%. This is in agreement with the large national program under way in Germany, where the Hemoccult II slide is being used. Our initial false-positive rate for neoplasia was 0.5% using the single Hemoccult slide. This has increased to 2.1% using the Hemoccult II slide but is offset by the higher yield of positive neoplasia results. The majority of patients have demonstrated one or two positive slides; rarely does a patient have five or six positive slides.

Asymptomatic cancers detected in both of the national programs appear to have favorable pathological staging, which supports the early observations of Greegor in this regard. The false-negative rate has yet to be established firmly but it is apparent that there are false negatives for adenomas and for cancer. The sensitivity of the slide test in detecting colorectal cancer in our series seems to be high, approximately 80%, and the false negativity 20%, but firm figures will have to await further follow-up of our screened group. It appears that the sensitivity for adenomas is of a much lower order of magnitude. Additional screening techniques should be used in conjunction with the fecal occult blood test, especially sigmoidoscopy, because of the lower sensitivity for adenomas and because of the false negatives for cancer.

APPROACH TO DIAGNOSIS AND SCREENING

When patients present with symptoms suggesting colonic disease, we must use all of our techniques to provide an accurate diagnosis, including sigmoidoscopy, air-contrast barium enema, and colonoscopy with biopsy and cytology. The aggressiveness of the workup will depend on the symptoms and the patient's risk factors. Earlier diagnosis in symptomatic patients may provide a more favorable prognosis. However, the best possible prognosis will occur in patients who are asymptomatic. Evidence suggests that we may expect a 15-year survival of 80 to 90% of such patients. Screening, therefore, should be applied to men and women over the age of 40 on an annual basis, these people being considered to be at standard risk for colorectal cancer. A reasonable approach to this group of patients may be fecal occult blood testing every year and sigmoidoscopy every three to five years. At the present time, sigmoidoscopy is being done by the rigid technique. The future role of flexible sigmoidoscopy remains to be determined. Patients who have a positive screening test should have an aggressive workup with air-contrast barium enema, colonoscopy, and biopsy and cytology when necessary.

Patients at risk because of known underlying premalignant disease such as ulcerative colitis over 7 years, or familial polyposis, must be screened directly, using roentgenography, endoscopy, and cytology on a periodic basis since occult blood testing is of no value in these groups. At the present time, we screen these patients every six months with sigmoidoscopy and every year with colonoscopy. Patients with a significant family history of colon cancer must have screening at an earlier age, beginning perhaps at age 21. In addition to fecal occult blood testing and sigmoidoscopy, we have to consider periodic testing with barium enema and colonoscopy in some of these groups of patients, such as those with familial cancer syndromes and site-specific hereditary colon cancer. Patients with a previous history of colonic polyps or colon cancer must have their colons cleared of synchronous lesions by roentgenography and colonoscopy and then have periodic examinations by these methods as well as occult blood testing annually.

Thus a significant reduction in colorectal cancer mortality and incidence could result if there is a reorientation of our approach to an early aggressive diagnostic study of symptomatic patients and screening of asymptomatic patients in our individual practices, clinics, and the community at large within the framework of cost-effectiveness.

If we are to make any significant change in the long-term survival of patients with colon cancer, we will have to take an aggressive position with screening and diagnostic techniques as outlined above. Patient compliance has been excellent when physicians present a positive attitude regarding the importance of early diagnosis. We now have all the techniques necessary for detection of early colon cancer if applied together in meaningful sequences. The use of these methods in aggressive programs coupled with increased public awareness could, over a period of years, increase the percentage of early lesions coming to surgery in a way analogous to that seen in Japan for gastric cancer, using roentgenogram and endoscopic techniques (44). Ideally, these programs should be incorporated into multiphasic screening approaches for cancer at multiple organ sites as well as other significant disease (12,45). Detection of adenomas is as important as detection of early colon cancer if we accept their relationship to cancer. If we can extrapolate from the experience of rectosigmoid polypectomy, colonic polypectomy could result in lower incidence of colon cancer in the population with adenomas if these patients have periodic surveillance for future lesions.

Many of these proposed approaches will have to be tested within the framework of controlled trials.

REFERENCES

1. Miller DG: The early diagnosis of cancer, in Homburger F (ed): *Physiopathology of Cancer.* Basel: S Karger, 1976, vol. 2, pp 5–64.

2. Balachandra VK, Schottenfeld D, Berg JW, Robbins GF: Patterns of delay and extent of disease in radical mastectomy patients, 1940–1943, 1950–1955, and 1960–1965. *Clin Bull* (Memorial Sloan-Kettering Cancer Center) 3:10–13, 1973.

3. Winawer SJ, Sherlock P, Schottenfeld D, Miller DG: Screening for colon cancer. *Gastroenterol* 70:783–789, 1976.

4. Winawer SJ, Leidner SD, Kurtz RC: Flexible sigmoidoscopy compared to other diagnostic techniques in the detection of colorectal cancer and polyps. *Gastrointest Endosc* 23:243, 1977.

5. Bohlman TW, Katon RM, Lipshutz GR, et al: Fiberoptic pansigmoidoscopy. An evaluation and comparison with rigid sigmoidoscopy. *Gastroenterol* 72: 644-649, 1977.

6. Miller RE: Detection of colon carcinoma and the barium enema. *JAMA* 230:1195-1198, 1974.

7. Williams CB, Hunt RH, Loose H, et al: Colonoscopy in the management of colon polyps. *Br J Surg* 61:673-682, 1974.

8. Winawer S, Weston E, Hajdu S, et al: Sensitivity of diagnostic techniques in patients with positive fecal occult blood screening tests. Presented at the Annual Meeting of the American Society for Gastrointestinal Endoscopy, Las Vegas (Nevada), May 24, 1978.

9. Overholt BF: Colonoscopy—a review. *Gastroenterol* 68:1308-1320, 1975.

10. Deddish MR, Hertz RE: Colotomy and coloscopy in the management of neoplasms of the colon. *Dis Colon Rectum* 2:133-138, 1959.

11. Winawer SJ, Leidner SD, Miller DG, et al: Results of a screening program for the detection of early colon cancer and polyps using fecal occult blood testing. *Gastroenterol* 72(5:2):A-127/1150, 1977.

12. Schottenfeld D: Patient risk factors and the detection of early colon cancer. *Prev Med* 1:335-351, 1972.

13. Winawer SJ, Leidner SD, Hajdu SI, et al: Colonoscopic biopsy and cytology in the diagnosis of colon cancer. *Cancer* 42:2849-2853, 1978.

14. '78 Cancer Facts and Figures. American Cancer Society, 1978.

15. Lynch HT, Guirgis H, Swartz M, et al: Genetics and colon cancer. *Arch Surg* 106:669-675, 1973.

16. Sherlock P, Lipkin M, Winawer SJ: Predisposing factors in colon carcinoma, in Stollerman, GH (ed): *Advances in Internal Medicine*. Chicago, Year Book Medical Publisher, Inc, 1975, vol 20, pp 121-150.

17. Edwards FC, Truelove SC: Course and prognosis of ulcerative colitis. IV. Carcinoma of the colon. *Gut* 5:1-22, 1964.

18. Morson BC: Cancer in ulcerative colitis. *Gut* 7:425-426, 1966.

19. Devroede GJ, Taylor WF, Sauer WG, et al: Cancer risk and life expectancy of children with ulcerative colitis. *N Engl J Med* 285:17-21, 1971.

20. Weedon DD, Shorter RG, Ilstrup DM, et al: Crohn's disease and cancer. *N Engl J Med* 289:1099-1103, 1973.

21. Hertz RE, Deddish MR, Day E: Value of periodic examination in detecting cancer of the rectum and colon. *Postgrad Med* 27:290-294, 1960.

22. Moertel CG, Hill JR, Dockerty MB: The routine proctoscopic examination: a second look. *Mayo Clin Proc* 41:368-374, 1966.

23. Wilson GS, Dale EH, Brines OA: An evaluation of polyps detected in 20,847 routine sigmoidoscope examinations. *Am J Surg* 90:834-840, 1955.

24. Bolt RJ: Sigmoidoscopy in detection and diagnosis in the asymptomatic individual. *Cancer* 28:121-122, 1971.

25. Hertz RE: The management of adenomas of the large gut, in Stearns MW Jr (ed): *Neoplasms of the Colon, Rectum, and Anus*. New York, John Wiley & Sons, 1980, pp 00-00.

26. Gilbertsen VA: Proctosigmoidoscopy and polypectomy in reducing the incidence of rectal cancer. *Cancer* 34:936-939, 1974.

27. Lennard-Jones JE, Morson BC, Ritchie JK, et al: Cancer in colitis: Assessment of the individual risk by clinical and histological criteria. *Gastroenterol* 73:1280-1289, 1977.

28. Morson BC: Genesis of colorectal cancer. *Clin Gastroenterol* 5:3:505-525, 1976.

29. Ostrow JD, Mulvaney CA, Hansel JR, Rhodes RS: Sensitivity and reproducibility of chemical tests for fecal occult blood with an emphasis on false-positive reactions. *Am J Dig Dis* 18:930-940, 1973.

30. Greegor DH: Occult blood testing for detection of asymptomatic colon cancer. *Cancer* 28:131-134, 1971.

31. Greegor DH: Diagnosis of large-bowel cancer in the asymptomatic patient. *JAMA* 201:943-945, 1967.

32. Glober GA, Peskoe SM: Outpatient screening for gastrointestinal lesions using guaiac-impregnated slides. *Am J Dig Dis* 19:399-403, 1974.

33. Hastings JB: Mass screening for colorectal cancer. *Am J Surg* 127:228-233, 1974.

34. Gnauck R: Screening for colorectal cancer using guaiac-slides (abstract). Third International Symposium on Detection and Prevention of Cancer, May 1976.

35. Miller RE: Detection of colon carcinoma and the barium enema. *JAMA* 230:1195, 1974.

36. Winawer SJ: Fecal occult blood testing. *Am J Dig Dis* 21:885–888, 1976.

37. Stroehlein JR, Fairbanks VF, McGill DB, Go VLW: Hemoccult detection of fecal blood quantitated by radioassay. *Am J Dig Dis* 21:841–844, 1976.

38. Ostrow JD, Mulvaney CA, Hansel JR, Rhodes RS: Sensitivity and reproducibility of chemical tests for fecal occult blood with an emphasis on false-positive reactions. *Am J Dig Dis* 18:930–940, 1973.

39. Fleisher M, Schwartz MK, Winawer SJ: The false-negative Hemoccult test. *Gastroenterol* 72:782–784, 1977.

40. Fleisher M, Schwartz MK, Winawer SJ: The use of fecal occult blood testing in detecting colorectal cancer. *Clin Chem* 23:1157, 1977.

41. Winawer S, Ginther M, Weston E, et al: Impact of modifications in fecal occult blood test on screening program for colorectal neoplasia. Presented at the Annual Meeting of the American Gastroenterological Association, Las Vegas (Nevada), May 23, 1978.

42. Greegor DH: Detection of colon cancer in the asymptomatic patient. Presented at the Third International Symposium on Detection and Prevention of Cancer, May, 1976.

43. Bond JH, Gilbertsen VA: Early detection of colonic carcinoma by mass screening for occult stool blood: preliminary report. *Gastroenterol* 72(5):A-8/1031, 1977.

44. Yamagata S, Masuda H, Oshiba S, et al: Epidemiology and symptomatology of early cancer of stomach, *Recent Advances of Gastroenterology,* Proceedings Third World Congress of Gastroenterology. Tokyo: Nankodo Co, vol 1, pp 487–489, 1967.

45. Lynch HT, Harlon W, Swartz M, et al: Multiphasic mobile cancer screening: a positive approach to early detection and control. *Cancer* 30:774–780, 1972.

3
Medical Considerations in the Surgical Management of Neoplasms of the Colon, Rectum, and Anus

Charles S. LaMonte

There are at least three constituents of the medical assessment of patients presenting for colorectal surgery: a thorough evaluation of the patient's medical conditions which may affect intraoperative or postoperative care; acquaintance with the surgical procedures being contemplated and with the risks and pathophysiologic consequences of each procedure; and investment in the improvement of remediable conditions and anticipation of probable or possible postoperative complications. From these considerations it is clear that the medical consultant will often be an essential active participant in the care of the surgical patient.

The corollary of such an active role for the internist is that neither the request for the consultation nor the service rendered can be perfunctory. Ideally the medical consultant, in complicated cases, should be included early in the planning of the patient's treatment. This treatment plan must make allowances for potential delay so that the internist can correct some preexisting medical abnormalities and present the candidate for surgery in optimum medical condition. It is important for the surgeon and for the medical consultant to develop a close collaborative relationship which clearly delineates the respective areas of responsibility, particularly as relates to writing orders. Finally, the medical consultant must expect continued active involvement in the course of the complicated patient. It is difficult to speak of any absolute contraindication to surgical management of colorectal cancer. The internist must be prepared to assume some of the responsibility and risks for operative management and may participate with the surgeon in attempting to balance these risks against the likely success or outcome of surgery.

EVALUATION OF THE PATIENT

The preceding considerations imply a comprehensive and thorough assessment of the patient's medical condition, especially the review of organ systems. Table 1 lists the medical conditions encountered by one internist consultant in 1713 evaluations of surgical patients. It must be recognized that this experience to some degree reflects the subspecialty interests of this consultant in cardiology and pulmonary disease. Therefore, there may

Table 1. Diagnostic Impression at Time of Consultation

	Colorectal (88 patients expressed in percent[a])	All Surgical (1,713 patients expressed in percent[a])
Cardiovascular		
Atherosclerotic heart disease	18	20
Hypertensive cardiovascular disease	15	13
Cardiomyopathy	—	1
Valvular lesion	2	3
Congenital abnormality	—	1
Congestive heart failure	5	2
Conduction defect	1	2
Arrhythmia	18	10
Pericardial disease	1	1
Syncope, cardiac arrest	2	1
Peripheral arterial disease	3	3
Peripheral venous disease	3	1
Abnormal electrocardiogram	2	3
Pacemaker	—	1
Hypotension, shock	—	1
Subacute bacterial endocarditis	—	0.4
Pulmonary emboli	1	1.1
Pulmonary		
Chronic obstructive pulmonary disease	8	14
Asthma	5	2
Interstitial disease	1	2
Pneumonia	1	2
Pulmonary insufficiency	2	1
Pleural disease	1	3
Prior tuberculosis	2	2
Other cancer	3	9
Endocrinology and Metabolism		
Endocrine disorder	3	1
Diabetes	9	6
Gout	1	2
Hypercalcemia	—	1
Nutritional deficiency	1	0.4
Obesity	1	1
Hyperlipidemia	—	0.3

Table 1. (Continued)

	Colorectal (88 patients expressed in percent[a])	All Surgical (1,713 patients expressed in percent[a])
Nephrology		
Prior renal dysfunction	3	2
Electrolyte abnormality	1	0.4
Neurology		
Prior cerebrovascular event	1	1
Parkinsonism	1	0.2
Other neurologic abnormality	2	3
Psychiatric condition	—	0.1
Gastroenterology		
Hepatic dysfunction	2	2
Other G.I. disorder	2	5
Allergy and infectious disease		
Infections	1	2
Allergic and autoimmune diseases	1	1
Arthritis	—	0.4
Hematologic disorder	—	1
Dermatologic condition	1	0.2
Glaucoma	—	0.5

[a] Totals exceed 100% because of occurrence of multiple conditions in several patients.

have been preselection of the patients referred for consultation. Second, it should be noted that the impression reflects the initial diagnostic impression. In many cases subsequent evaluation of the patient has disclosed additional or different diagnoses. However, no data are readily available to correct for this possibility. Finally, not all of these 1713 patients were seen preoperatively, and some of the consultations may have been requested for complications in the postoperative period. This variable has not been corrected in the presentation of the data. Nevertheless, there is merit to a review of these various medical considerations. Certainly the table reflects the wide variety of medical complications or potential complications in the surgical population. It therefore indicates the relative importance of the portions of the review of systems which the consulting internist should conduct. Some specific comments concerning these areas of medical subspecialty are in order.

MEDICAL SUBSPECIALTIES

Cardiovascular Disease

From the point of view of the surgeon and the anesthesiologist, cardiovascular disease may be the most important medical consideration in the preoperative evaluation of the surgical patient. In the age group at risk for colorectal carcinoma, atherosclerotic heart disease constitutes the major category. The consulting internist must correlate the clinical history and physical examination with the routine electrocardiogram. Particularly troublesome in the experience at Memorial Hospital has been equivocal Q waves in leads II, III, AVF, V5, and V6, or the poor progression of R waves in leads V_1 through V_3. In general, confronted with equivocal laboratory data, the medical consultants have tended to rely most heavily on clinical history and physical findings.

An area of special concern is the relatively small group of patients in whom a prosthetic cardiac valve has been implanted. In this group the surgeon has a particular responsibility to include the internist or cardiologist at an early stage of treatment planning. The perioperative management of the patient's anticoagulation is a critical concern that requires close coordination of the medical and surgical teams.

Along with prosthetic valves, intrinsic valvular lesions and implanted devices such as cardiac pacemakers necessitate planning for antibiotic prophylaxis. The internist, of course, recognizes the murmurs of aortic valve deformity and mitral stenosis. Because of its subtlety and variability, the internist must be alert to the late systolic click syndrome of mitral valve prolapse, or Barlow's syndrome, which is also associated with a high incidence of subacute bacterial endocarditis and requires antibiotic prophylaxis during colorectal surgery. Other congenital cardiovascular lesions such as patent ductus arteriosus, atrial septal defect, or pulmonic stenosis also require antibiotic prophylaxis.

Of particular concern regarding the cardiovascular status of the preoperative patient with colorectal carcinoma is the possibility or risk of congestive heart failure in the postoperative state. This has been a major consideration of the medical consultant and constitutes a focus of the history, careful physical examination, and assessment of the chest x-ray film. The risk of congestive heart failure frequently warrants specialized studies, which in our institution have included assessment of "physiologic parameters" by means of Swan-Ganz catheterization of the pulmonary artery and determination of cardiac output.

Of greater applicability and clinical availability is the information obtained from echocardiography. Not only is this information pertinent to some of the considerations discussed above, particularly in the areas of rheumatic deformity of the aortic or mitral valve, congenital bicuspid aortic valve, and mitral valve prolapse, but it is also particularly valuable in evaluating left ventricular function and performance. Although the experience at Memorial Hospital with echocardiography is of short duration, it is proving a fruitful and reliable special diagnostic procedure. It has wider applicability than does stress electrocardiography in the assessment of physiology and function. However, stress testing has frequently been valuable in clarifying the cause of atypical chest pains suggestive of angina pectoris.

Hypertensive cardiovascular disease is another frequently encountered cardiac condition in the group of patients presenting for colorectal surgery. It should be noted that the blood pressure as recorded immediately after the patient's admission to the hospital is invariably elevated and should not necessarily be accepted as the patient's true value. Usually, the patient has been diagnosed before admission to have hypertension and may already be on a very satisfactory medical regimen. With the various drugs, however, the side effects must be assessed and the implications for operative and postoperative management must be determined. Specifically, the hypokalemia accompanying diuretic therapy and the potential for cardiac decompensation associated with propranalol therapy deserve mention. At Memorial Hospital, the preoperative administration of alpha methyldopa and reserpine has not resulted in any intraoperative difficulty. Any associated hypotension after anesthesia induction is readily managed by plasma colloid replacement. Usually the patients presenting in this surgical group are not at risk for pheochromocytoma, and detailed preoperative evaluation has not been performed. However, the internist must be aware of this diagnostic possibility and must not hesitate, when there is strong clinical suspicion, to defer surgery until there has been a conclusive diagnostic workup.

Another area of cardiovascular concern relates to disease of peripheral arteries. The internist should particularly document the patency of the carotid arteries and also the presence of a pulse on the four extremities. Despite attention to this matter, there have been instances of postoperative thrombosis, particularly in the iliofemoral circulation. The cerebral vascular circulation and possible carotid artery stenosis are of particular importance in the anesthetic management of the patient during intubation.

Cardiac arrhythmias often are functional, related to supratentorial influences on the sympathetic nervous system. It is important to try to distinguish whether ectopic beats reflect such extracardiac influences or whether they are a sign of intracardiac disease. In the latter case, and/or at the request of the anesthesiologist, appropriate treatment as indicated below may be necessary.

Finally, a particular search must be made for evidence of intracardiac conduction defect. The existence of a diseased sinoatrial node or of bifascicular intraventricular block may mandate preoperative pacemaker insertion as discussed below.

Pulmonary Disease

If cardiovascular disease is a conspicuous concern in the preoperative period, pulmonary disease may represent the most underrecognized medical abnormality. Such omissions occur with obstructive pulmonary disease, interstitial processes, and pneumoconiosis but are not likely to be true of asthma, which is, in itself, a relatively dramatic disease process and tends to reside in demonstrative individuals.

A history of tobacco abuse or of industrial exposure should alert the internist to the possibility of obstructive pulmonary disease or pneumoconiosis. Similarly, in the assessment of exercise tolerance there may be clues to the existence of either obstructive or interstitial disease. The chest roentgenogram, though often helpful, frequently fails to indicate these entities. The patient's history and symptoms are usually a more reliable guide to their presence.

Especially in the postoperative period, earlier recognition of lung diseases is crucial and may determine the outcome of the patient's hospital course. Formal pulmonary function testing, to include not only spirometry but especially arterial blood analysis, provides the criterion and essential baseline for postoperative management. Because diffuse pulmonary disease is radiographically so subtle and often inapparent, and because the patient's history and physical examination may be difficult to assess, the internist should be particularly ready to suggest such formal pulmonary function testing preoperatively.

Endocrinology and Metabolism

This is a significant albeit subtle area of concern. The most frequent condition is that of glucose intolerance. A prior history of diabetes or an elevated blood glucose upon admission are the obvious clues. It is fruitful to attempt preoperatively to determine the renal threshold for glucose, since the postoperative management of the diabetic patient entails treatment of glycosuria by insulin coverage. If the patient is on fractional urines preoperatively, frequently this renal threshold can be determined by means of a blood glucose drawn when the patient spills trace or 1+ glycosuria. Alternatively, a glucose tolerance test may be indicated.

Of concern especially among patients with neoplastic disease is the possibility of hypercalcemia. As noted in Table 1, this was not encountered among patients with operable colorectal carcinoma. It is not uncommon among the patients with broncho-genic carcinoma or carcinoma of the urinary bladder. If it is detected in the patient with colorectal carcinoma, hypercalcemia mandates an evaluation for metastatic disease, or identification of another explanation for the abnormality.

Possible abnormalities of thyroid and/or adrenal function constitute a significant but subtle area of concern. If undetected in the preoperative state, such abnormalities may contribute to alarming and mysterious postoperative difficulties. Other than evaluating serum electrolytes, physiognomy, and body build, screening for adrenal dysfunction is probably not feasible. The awareness of skin temperature and moisture, of eye motions and appearance, and of spontaneous level of activity may provide insights to thyroid dys-function. If a deficiency of thyroid and/or adrenal activity is suspected, the possibility of an underlying pituitary abnormality and panhypopituitarism should be assessed.

Nephrology

Assessment of the renal function preoperatively, at least by means of serum creatinine rather than level of urea nitrogen, is mandatory in the management of colorectal cancer. In anticipation of the need for aminoglycoside or other potentially nephrotoxic drug therapy, it is frequently important to measure the creatinine clearance. Management of lesions of the cecum, sigmoid colon, or rectum necessitates intravenous pyelography. A history of recurrent urinary tract infections, symptoms of bladder outlet obstruction, or prior occurrence of renal calculi should be noted. Finally, the patient's serum electrolyte status must be documented, especially when there has been diarrhea, either spontaneous or induced in the bowel preparation.

Neurology

Often it is not necessary to conduct a formal assessment of the patient's neurologic status. During the remainder of the medical evaluation, the patient's speech pattern, motions, and behavior will alert the internist to potential problems or complications. Items of specific concern, however, ought to be noted and/or excluded. The existence of Parkinsonism carries significant implications for the anesthetic management and for postoperative respiratory care. The presence of any neuropathy or myopathy may also be significant in the postoperative state. Finally, frequently encountered, but seldom explicitly acknowledged, are abnormalities in the mental status of the patient. Particu-larly among the elderly there may be dementia, which will impair the patient's coopera-tion in the postoperative period, when his active participation is crucial to the avoidance of such complications as atelectasis, pneumonitis, and thrombophlebitis. Of lesser importance in the author's experience is the presence of prior cerebral vascular accident and hemiparesis. This condition arouses concern, as it may indicate underlying systemic disease such as hypertensive cardiovascular disease or peripheral atherosclerosis.

Gastroenterology

In this subspecialty, the most important concern for the internist is the adequacy of hepatic function. The review of systems should include explicit inquiry about prior hepatitis or jaundice. The physical examination must include a search for splenomegaly, telangiectasia, palmar erythema, and other stigmata of chronic hepatocellular disease. Among laboratory data possible hyperglobulinemia or depression of prothrombin time are important. The history of prior peptic ulcer disease should be determined, in order to anticipate any tendency postoperatively to upper gastrointestinal bleeding. Similarly, the existence of biliary tract disease and recurrent pancreatitis must be documented.

Miscellaneous

Because of their infrequency, discussion of abnormalities in the subspecialty areas of allergy and infectious disease, hematology, rheumatology, and dermatology does not seem warranted. In most centers the routine laboratory workup includes determination of the platelet count, prothrombin time, and activated partial thromboplastin time. When these procedures are not part of the mandated admission evaluation of patients, they should be specifically requested.

RISKS OF THE PROCEDURES

The medical consultant must consider particularly the risks associated with the proposed colorectal surgery. It is only in terms of this awareness that he can most appropriately prepare for the postoperative course and patient management. In addition this awareness will intensify the consultant's evaluation of or search for specific medical considerations.

The likelihood of bacteremia during surgery focuses attention on possible valvular cardiac disease, mitral valve prolapse, certain congenital cardiac lesions, and implanted devices such as prosthetic valves and pacemakers.

The possibility of blood volume instability because of a loss of plasma volume into third space is an especially important consideration. The internist must have anticipated the risks which may be associated with episodes of hypotension, with need for pressor or cardiotonic drug therapy, and with possible fluid overload. These considerations focus critical attention on the cardiovascular system.

A third area of predictable difficulty is the inhibition of ventilation after extensive abdominal incision and surgical manipulation. The reduction of vital capacity and of measures of forced expiratory flow is well documented in the immediate postoperative period. This fact directs particular attention to respiratory training and preparation preoperatively.

Despite the commitment of a well-equipped and well-staffed institution to the most effective, and therefore usually the most aggressive, mode of therapy, some patients are unable to tolerate surgery. Certainly patients in Class IV of the New York Heart Association classification, and patients with pulmonary disease of comparable severity, should be considered inoperable. For other patients, discussion and close cooperation between surgical and medical teams may permit a modification of the surgical plan to offer the patient the most effective therapy permissible. The results of such treatment, determined through close collaboration and negotiation, can be gratifying.

PREOPERATIVE PREPARATION

From the preceding discussion, the imperative to correct potentially remediable medical conditions is obvious. The most significant ones are listed in Table 2. A few selective comments are in order.

Regarding recognized atherosclerotic cardiovascular disease, published data indicate that myocardial infarction occurring more than six months before surgery increases the risk of surgery relatively little. Similarly, the existence of stable angina pectoris increases the risk, but irreducibly so. However, there has been a disturbing frequency of asymptomatic myocardial infarction between admission to Memorial Hospital and performance of surgery. Frequently the recording of a second electrocardiogram immediately prior to surgery has disclosed the interval myocardial insult. Although the author does not recommend routine performance of repeated electrocardiograms preoperatively, the value in selected situations is noted. At least the importance of a medical reevaluation of the patient after a prolonged workup and just before surgery is recommended. Patients with recognized atherosclerotic heart disease undergo routine intraoperative and postoperative cardiac monitoring at our hospital. In addition, we obtain a routine electrocardiogram in the postoperative period to be certain that there has been no silent interval myocardial infarction.

The need for correction of any antecedent congestive heart failure and for vigilance for its occurrence in the postoperative state is obvious. Patients with hypertension have

Table 2. Conditions Which May Require Preoperative Correction or Control

Cardiovascular
  Hypertension
  Congestive heart failure
  Some arrhythmias
Pulmonary
  Chronic obstructive pulmonary disease
  Asthma
Endocrinology and metabolism
  Diabetes
  Gout
  Adrenal or thyroid insufficiency
Nephrology
  Electrolyte imbalance
Gastroenterology
  Hepatic dysfunction
Hematology
  Anemia
  Thrombocytopenia
  Deficiency of coagulation factors

usually been diagnosed prior to their admission for treatment of colorectal carcinoma. However, occasionally patients admitted for such surgery have undetected and severe hypertension which requires preoperative treatment. It has been the practice at Memorial Hospital to use a combination of diuretics, antiadrenergic agents, and vasodilators that can be administered intravenously during the postoperative period. The specific drugs commonly employed are furosemide, alpha methyldopa, and hydralazine.

Patients with partially reversible chronic obstructive pulmonary disease often benefit from an interval of preoperative physical therapy and bronchodilator treatments. The investment in physical therapy and rehabilitative medicine is particularly important in view of the frequent association of postoperative pulmonary embarrassment with colorectal surgery. Among the many pharmacologic agents available the author favors a progressive approach beginning with aerosol delivery of a beta 2 sympathomimetic agent such as isoetharine delivered via motor nebulizer. In addition to bronchodilatation, this preoperative treatment enhances sputum mobilization and production. The second step of pharmacologic intervention is oral administration of a theophylline compound, which can be continued via the intravenous route in the postoperative period. Third, it may be necessary to administer systemically a beta 2 agonist such as terbutaline, which has the advantage that it also can be administered subcutaneously when the patient is in the nonabsorptive state. Caution must be exercised, however, with administration of terbutaline, which can cause significant tachycardia or hypertension. Among patients with obstructive pulmonary disease, especially the chronic bronchitics with purulent sputum, preoperative sputum culture for antibiotic sensitivity is worthwhile.

For patients with diabetes mellitus, the importance of ascertaining the renal threshold for glucose has already been mentioned. Among such patients with a normal renal threshold around 160 to 180 mg%, insulin coverage can conveniently be administered by means of a sliding scale. In patients with a high renal threshold it may be necessary to plan postoperative management of the diabetes by means of periodic blood glucose determinations.

The importance of preoperative identification of hepatocellular disease and dysfunction cannot be overemphasized. When suspected, this abnormality may influence the choice of antibiotic in the preoperative bowel preparation so as to sterilize the gut to prevent urea cleavage and ammonia retention. Kanamycin is frequently routinely employed in the bowel preparation and is appropriate in this situation. Neomycin is another commonly used drug. In the postoperative period, the patient must be closely observed for evidence of encephalopathy, and provision of maximum carbohydrate calories by intravenous infusion should be assured.

Deficiency of coagulation factors will routinely be disclosed by means of the screening laboratory tests mentioned previously. Thrombocytopenia must be explained and corrected whenever possible. If a specific cause such as idiopathic thrombocytopenic purpura cannot be identified and treated, transfusion of fresh pooled platelets to achieve a platelet count exceeding 75,000 is in order. In the hypoprothrombinemic state, assuming that this abnormality is not iatrogenic, administration of vitamin K orally or parenterally is indicated. Coagulation disorders persisting after vitamin K administration usually respond to administration of fresh frozen plasma.

Among several groups of patients, correction of the condition before surgery is not possible. These patients should be aware of the risks associated with extensive abdominal surgery; and the importance of preoperative training in effective respiration, cough maneuvers, and general physical activity must be stressed. Such conditions include disorientation, dementia, neuromuscular deficiency, Parkinsonism, and irreversible chronic obstructive pulmonary disease. In addition, among patients with Parkinson's disease, the importance of avoiding parasympathomimetic drugs such as edrophonium and bethanechol is noted. Finally, the possible benefit of parasympatholytic agents is apparent.

DIFFICULT MANAGEMENT DECISIONS

There are four conditions for which the course of management is not presently clearly indicated: antibiotic prophylaxis, maintenance of stable cardiac rhythm, anticoagulation, and high-risk coronary arterial disease. These will be discussed in the following paragraphs.

Antibiotic Prophylaxis

When recognized, there are certain obvious indications for antibiotic prophylaxis in patients undergoing colorectal surgery. The most common one is valvular cardiac disease, usually rheumatic or atherosclerotic deformity of the mitral and/or aortic valves. The recommendations of the American Heart Association Committee on the Prevention of Bacterial Endocarditis apply. At Memorial Hospital the regimen of choice is a combination of intravenous ampicillin and gentamycin. Our procedure is to administer gentamycin in a dose of 1.5 mg per kg up to 80 mg within the hour preceding surgery and every 8 hours thereafter for a total of at least 3 days. For patients not sensitive to penicillin and derivatives, ampicillin is administered 1 g intravenously within the hour prior to surgery and every 4 to 6 hr thereafter for at least 3 days. For patients allergic to penicillin, vancomycin is administered in a dose of 1 g over 30 min during the hour preceding surgery and erythromycin 500 mg every 6 hr for 3 days postoperatively.

Often, patients who are candidates for colon resection may have implanted cardiac pacemakers. These devices also mandate antibiotic prophylaxis as outlined above for valvular cardiac lesions.

Occasionally patients in the older age group possess congenital cardiac lesions. Infrequently one may encounter patients with interatrial septal defect, patent ductus arteriosus, or interventricular septal defect. These abnormalities likewise require antibiotic prophylaxis as outlined above. In patients with a systolic ejection murmur, the question whether or not there is valvular deformity is difficult. Echocardiography may distinguish among asymmetric septal hypertrophy, which does not call for antibiotic prophylaxis, and congenital bicuspid aortic valve or valvular deformity from other causes, which should be treated with antibiotic prophylaxis.

The consulting internist should be particularly alert to the possibility of the syndrome of late systolic click and murmur. Increasingly this congenital or developmental abnormality is recognized; it has a prevalence of perhaps 5% in a random adult population. Similarly, because of the predisposition of this lesion to subacute bacterial endocarditis, antibiotic prophylaxis is indicated. The dilemma for the internist is the subtlety and the variability of this cardiac lesion. The major challenge is detection of the problem, not determination of the appropriate course of management.

Stability of the Cardiac Rhythm

Many consultations for preoperative patients are requested because of cardiac arrhythmias. The problem is further complicated by the realization that many cases of ectopic beats have functional causes, particularly the tension and anxiety over admission to the hospital for resection of a probable malignancy. In particular, supraventricular ectopic beats generally should cause little concern. If they are relatively infrequent, simple observation is usually adequate. For frequent ectopic supraventricular beats, prophylactic digitalization against the possibility of a tachyarrhythmia such as atrial fibrillation is the most prudent course of action.

The problem of aberrantly conducted premature complexes is particularly frustrating. A significant proportion of such beats are aberrantly conducted junctional beats. Frequently ventricular ectopic complexes may reflect some subclinical congestive heart failure. Among the internists and cardiologists at Memorial Hospital, unifocal aberrantly conducted beats are considered relatively benign. If a fixed coupling interval between the antecedent normal complex and the ectopic complex can be established, the patient may be managed simply by expectant observation and preparedness to administer lidocaine bolus. On the other hand, if there is a variable coupling interval, or particularly if there are apparently multifocal ventricular premature complexes, the internist may elect either to digitalize the patient or to institute antiarrhythmic treatment with procainamide. Needless to say, the possibility of electrolyte disturbances or other metabolic abnormalities must be excluded.

A more subtle and controversial area concerns fascicular block of intraventricular conduction. Intraventricular block of a single fascicle should cause no concern. However, the presence of bifascicular block is disturbing and raises the threat of progression intraoperatively or immediately postoperatively to complete heart block. The current literature is inconclusive on this subject. However, a consensus is developing that anterior bifascicular block infrequently progresses to complete heart block. In such patients, it has not been the practice at Memorial Hospital routinely to insert a prophylactic temporary pacemaker catheter. Similarly, in complete left-bundle branch block, pacemaker catheters have not been utilized.

On the other hand, in a middle aged or elderly patient, the presence of a sinus bradycardia that does not respond to exercise warrants consideration of prophylactic pacemaker catheter insertion. Depending upon the accompanying cardiac findings the author favors preoperative insertion of such devices. The author also favors use of a prophylactic pacemaker catheter for significant atrioventricular conduction abnormality that cannot be attributed to digitalis or other drug or metabolic derangement, and for right-bundle branch block and left posterior hemiblock.

Indications for Anticoagulation

At this time there is considerable controversy about prophylactic minidose heparinization for prophylaxis of venous thrombosis. The author does not wish to endorse one view or the other. In patients undergoing simple colonic resection, he would not currently recommend such prophylactic heparinization. However, in a patient undergoing abdominal perineal resection, who may be immobilized for a longer period of time, the use of subcutaneous heparin, 5,000 units every 12 hours seems prudent.

There is another group of patients for whom documentation of the benefit of heparinization does not exist. However, the use of heparin seems warranted because of the dire consequences if thrombosis should occur. Among patients who have undergone coronary bypass surgery, for protection of this graft, the author favors subtherapeutic heparinization for 7 to 10 days. The same recommendation is made also for patients with evidence of cerebral vascular disease and/or carotid artery stenosis. For peripheral arterial disease involving the extremities, though the consequences of thrombosis are less catastrophic than in the two preceding situations, the author favors subtherapeutic heparinization. Finally, in the occasional patient who may present with thrombocytosis, antithrombotic measures seem warranted and the author recommends heparinization until aspirin and/or dipyridamole can be instituted. It should be emphasized that the preceding indications for anticoagulation are controversial and should be accepted only tentatively at the present time.

Management of Patients with Prosthetic Cardiac Valve

Occasionally a patient with previous implantation of a prosthetic cardiac valve requires colorectal surgery. The surgeon must appreciate the need for early involvement of the internist/consultant because these patients invariably are receiving chronic anticoagulation therapy. The strategy employed at our hospital is to terminate the Coumadin anticoagulant after the dose 72 hours prior to surgery. By 24 hr prior to surgery, the prothrombin time has usually returned nearly to normal levels. At this point, heparin infusion to maintain the partial thromboplastin time at approximately 60 sec is initiated and maintained until an hour prior to surgery. The heparin infusion is resumed approximately 2 hr after completion of surgery and is maintained until oral anticoagulation can be reinstituted.

Occasionally a patient whose Coumadin treatment has been suspended 72 hours before surgery may not completely correct the hypoprothrombinemic state. In such cases, fresh frozen plasma can be administered at the time of surgery. It should be emphasized that these patients likewise require antibiotic prophylaxis as outlined in the preceding section on valvular cardiac lesions.

Unstable Angina Pectoris, Recent Myocardial Infarction

In this group of patients, the risk of surgery clearly is markedly increased and the benefits from colon resection must be weighed critically against the risks of cardiovascular complication and/or death. The use of long-acting nitroglycerin, either as sublingual isosorbide or as nitroglycerin ointment, is most helpful just before the operation. Propranalol is avoided because of the adverse hemodynamic effect intraoperatively and because of the difficulty and risk of administering parenteral propranalol while the patient is nonabsorptive. In addition, the risk of rebound symptoms of cardiac ischemia with interruption of the propranalol must be considered. Among such patients in whom control of the angina can be achieved and surgery successfully accomplished, there is high risk of postoperative angina pectoris and possible myocardial infarction. Postoperative monitoring in the intensive care unit should be anticipated and the use of long-acting nitrates and subtherapeutic heparinization postoperatively should be planned.

Another related problem taxing the internist's judgment is the occurrence of an acute myocardial infarction during the six-month period preceding the date of planned surgery.

Although the work of Goldman et al (2) has demonstrated the increased risk of surgery in this period, one must recognize the certain outcome of an indefinite or imprudent postponement of surgery. In this quandary, surgery is permissible, possibly as early as two months after the myocardial infarction. If surgery is undertaken at such an earlier interval, it is mandatory to carefully monitor pulmonary artery and wedge pressures by Swan-Ganz catheter, to determine serum levels of creatine phosphokinase and its isoenzymes, and to record serial electrocardiograms. Such patients should be monitored in the intensive care unit and should be treated with prophylactic heparinizaton.

POSTOPERATIVE CARE

Ideally, the medical consultants will have anticipated the problems which may arise in the postoperative period. The preceding discussion has already indicated the areas of concern: surveillance of renal function, close observation of control of diabetes mellitus, maintenance of electrolyte balance, surveillance for possible myocardial infarction, treatment of possible reversible obstructive pulmonary disease, and avoidance of congestive heart failure.

In addition to conditions already noted for postoperative surveillance, the medical consultant must be particularly alert to two frequent complications. The first is maintenance of adequate, effective mechanisms for ventilation and cough. It is important in all patients undergoing major abdominal surgery, but especially among those with identified pulmonary disease or neuromuscular disorders, to continue the physical medicine and therapy regimen initiated in the preoperative period. Aside from personal supervision by nursing staff, respiratory therapists, and physical therapists, the patient should be encouraged to use incentive inspiratory devices whenever possible. Only in unusual circumstances has the use of intermittent positive pressure breathing been suggested.

A final area of recurrent concern is that of fluid replacement. The occurrence of fluid overload and congestive heart failure has been alluded to above. In the experience of this hospital, this iatrogenic maneuver accounts for the majority of postoperative dyspnea and/or deterioration of arterial oxygen tensions. Arterial hypoxemia is probably due to pulmonary congestion several times more frequently than it reflects pulmonary embolization. Nevertheless, these and other postoperative complications do occur. There is no substitute for the continuing critical observations and analysis of the medical/surgical team as such questions arise.

REFERENCES

1. Kaplan EL, et al: AHA committee report. Prevention of bacterial endocarditis. *Circulation* 56:139A, 1977.

2. Goldman L, et al: Multifactorial index of cardiac risk in noncardiac surgical procedures. *New Engl J Med* 297:845, 1977.

3. Redding JS, Yakaitis RW: Predicting the need for ventilatory assistance. *Maryland State Med J* 19:52, 1970.

4. Pastore JO, et al: The risk of advanced heart block in surgical patients with right bundle branch block and left axis deviation. *Circulation* 57:677, 1978.

5. Dhingra RC, et al: Chronic right bundle branch block and left posterior hemiblock. Clinical, electrophysiologic, and prognostic observations. *Am J Cardiol* 36:867, 1975.

6. Bigger JT Jr, et al: Ventricular arrhythmias in ischemic heart disease: Mechanism, prevalence, significance, and management. *Progr Cardiovasc Dis* 19:255, 1977.

7. Rosen KM, et al: Electrophysiologic significance of first degree atrioventricular block with intraventricular conduction disturbance. *Circulation* 43:491, 1971.

8. Scanlon PJ, Prior R, Blount SG, Jr: Right bundle branch block associated with left superior or inferior intraventricular block. *Circulation* 42:1123, 1970.

4

Pathological Aspects of Colon and Anorectal Cancer

Stephen S. Sternberg

INTRODUCTION

The majority of cancers of the large intestines are adenocarcinomas, and most are diagnosed with considerable accuracy, either by physical examination of the patient (rectal palpation and sigmoidoscopy) or by barium enema. Biopsy of lesions in the anal and rectosigmoid regions are frequently obtained for confirmation of the clinical impression. In instances where the lesion is more proximal, the appropriate operation is performed without biopsy confirmation when the roentgenographic appearance of the tumor is typical.

Rarely is there a diagnostic problem in terms of interpretation of a biopsy of the usual colonic adenocarcinoma. The rarely occurring anaplastic adenocarcinomas, the in situ carcinomas, and the infiltrating carcinomas noted in relatively small polyps are the types that offer difficulties. The importance of accurate interpretation of adequately sampled tissue cannot be overemphasized, in particular when an abdominoperineal resection may be the appropriate operative procedure. The surgeon and pathologist should discuss the case together, with the biopsy material at hand, whenever the identification of the lesion is not clear.

Compared to polyps and adenocarcinomas, other types of tumors of the large intestines are infrequent. Carcinoids occur much less often than in the appendix and small intestines. Of the soft tissue tumors, tumors of smooth muscle are probably of most importance. Lipomas, nerve tumors, and vascular tumors are rare. The carcinomas of the anorectal region and melanomas have features peculiar to that anatomic site and are discussed separately.

POLYPS

It is likely that most, if not all, adenocarcinomas of the large bowel arise in polyps having an adenomatous pattern, or at least in abnormal mucosa with adenomatous features. The so-called adenomatous polyp has a tubular growth pattern, whereas the villous adenoma has delicate frond-like protrusions. These patterns are often intermixed in the same polyp, and it is now generally recognized that these two types of polyps are not as

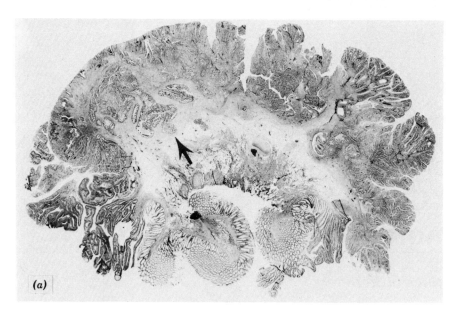

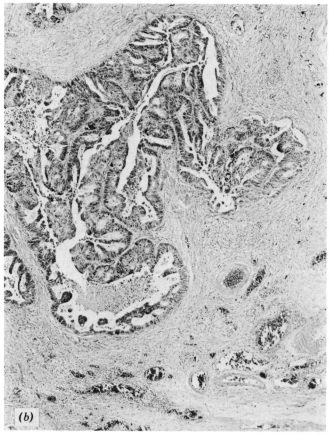

Figure 1. (*a*) Example of unequivocal adenocarcinoma arising in a polyp. The arrow indicates level of penetration [see parts (*b*) and (*c*)]. (*b*) infiltrating adenocarcinoma extending below muscularis mucosa. This is a higher magnification of the region near the arrow in part (*a*). (*c*) Individual adenocarcinomatous glands. [Compare to the glands illustrated under misplaced epithelium, Fig. 2(*c*).]

38

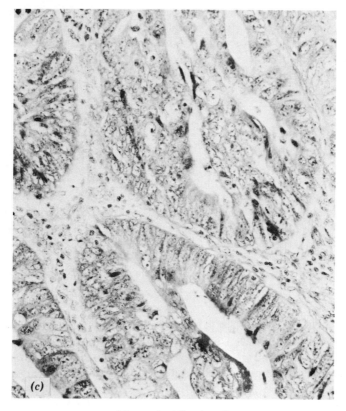

Figure 1. (*Continued*)

easily separable as pathologists were often obliged to indicate (1). Both villous and adenomatous polyps, or polyps showing features of both, can give rise to an adenocarcinoma. Hyperplastic (or metaplastic), inflammatory (or lymphoid), and hamartomatous polyps are not recognized as precursors of cancer.

Adenomatous polyps are much more common than the villous type. Villous tumors, however, are usually larger than the adenomatous type and more often have a cancer arising within them. Villous tumors have a predilection for the distal colon (rectosigmoid and rectum). Adenomatous polyps with villous features have a greater incidence of cancer than pure adenomatous polyps (1). The villous (or papillary) adenomas predominate in the rectosigmoid region. Invasive cancer in one series (215 cases) was found in 27% (2). Ninety percent were sessile; adenomatous polyps, on the other hand, are frequently pedunculated.

The lymphatic and capillary distribution in normal colon and in polyps has been examined by Fenoglio et al (3). Their studies provide a logical explanation for the failure to find lymphatic metastases in intramucosal carcinomas. The lymphatic vessels are associated with the base of the crypts and go no higher, even in the architectural distortion found in polyps. Only when the cancer approximates or involves the muscularis mucosa can lymphatic permeation occur. Of considerable importance in terms of treatment is the fact that small cancers of the type described assume a serious portent only if they are poorly differentiated (3,4). Well-differentiated carcinomas arising in polyps and showing invasion but no lymphatic permeation and containing a free stalk, can be considered cured by polypectomy (5) with rare exceptions (6) (Fig. 1).

Needless to say, when a polypectomy is performed in which there is present a superficially infiltrating carcinoma, or a segmental resection is the initial or subsequent treatment for a similar lesion, the specimens cannot be given a Dukes' classification. Without an examination of the full thickness of the bowel wall and of the regional lymph nodes, a Dukes' classification cannot be made.

MISPLACED EPITHELIUM

Pseudocarcinomatous Invasion, Adenomatous Polyp with Submucosal Cysts

This lesion has been adequately described by several authors (7–9), yet we continually observe instances where this lesion is confused microscopically with carcinoma in a polyp with invasion of the stalk. The lesion occurs less often than a true carcinoma in a polyp (2.4% in the series reported by Muto et al (7); about two times as many cancers in a polyp were seen in the same series). In another series where 21 polyps were found retrospectively to have misplaced epithelium, 18 were initially considered to be malignant (8). A large number of these polyps have a long stalk (75% at least 3 cm) and none were less than 1 cm.

The microscopic features appear as follows. (1) There is adenomatous epithelium beneath the muscularis mucosa, with the individual glands often dilated or cystic. (2) The glands show no more atypia than glands located above the muscularis; that is, other than the location, there are no features of carcinoma. (3) There are hemosiderin deposits in the stalk (Figs. 2 and 3). These three features are the most important in distinguishing misplacement from carcinomatous invasion. Further, there is no desmoplasia. It has been suggested that the long stalk, subject to twisting, results in hemorrhage and hemosiderin deposits.

NODULAR LYMPHOID HYPERPLASIA

This lesion is not precancerous, nor does it ordinarily present as a diagnostic problem in terms of biopsy interpretation. However, there have been several tragic cases of unnecessary colectomy as a result of misinterpretation of biopsy material. Nodular lymphoid hyperplasia can mimic familial polyposis, both endoscopically and roentgenographically. Misreading from an indadequate biopsy (or one that is superficial, or not containing lymphoid tissue), or interpreting a few irregular glands as adenomatous, can and has resulted in unnecessary surgery (10–13) *The diagnosis of "adenomatous polyp" is a serious one and can result in a colectomy.*

ADENOCARCINOMA OF COLON AND RECTUM

Gross Examination in the Pathology Laboratory of Large Bowel Cancer

Colon and rectal specimens are described in the fresh state. If time permits, several hours of fixation will facilitate the cutting of sections. Whether or not the orientation in regard to proximal or distal is known, the distance from the tumor to both ends of the specimen should be indicated. We divide the lymph nodes into three groups: the lymph nodes proximal to the tumor make up level I, those opposite the tumor, level II, and those distal to the tumor, level III. The highest lymph node is usually sent as a separate specimen by the surgeon. The tumor must be amply sampled, keeping in mind three points, namely, that sections are to show the (1) type of tumor and grade, (2) continuity with normal mucosa or polypoid tissue and in situ changes, and (3) the deepest penetration in the wall. Other sections should include both margins of resections, which will also show the condition of the nontumorous mucosa. Any other abnormalities in the specimen should, of course, also be sampled for microscopic examination such as polyps and diverticuli. *All* lymph nodes in the specimen should be dissected out and submitted for microscopic examination.

In regard to margins, the pathologist should realize that considerable contraction of tissues occur from the time the tumor is in situ until sections are taken for microscopic

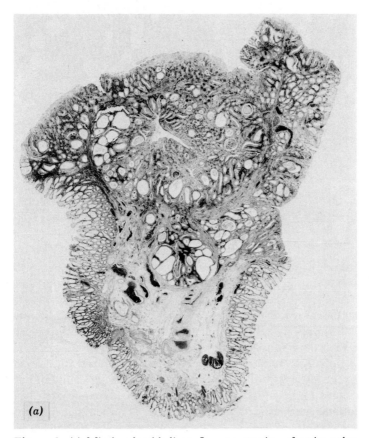

(a)

Figure 2. (a) Misplaced epithelium. Low-power view of entire polyp (8×), showing bulk of epithelium beneath muscularis mucosa. (b) Example of misplaced epithelium that may be mistaken for infiltrating carcinoma [same polyp as in part (a)]. Epithelium present beneath muscularis mucosa; portion of adenomatous polyp at upper right. Note hemosiderin in stroma, a characteristic feature. (c) Higher power shows glands with only minimal atypia; compare to Figure 1(c).

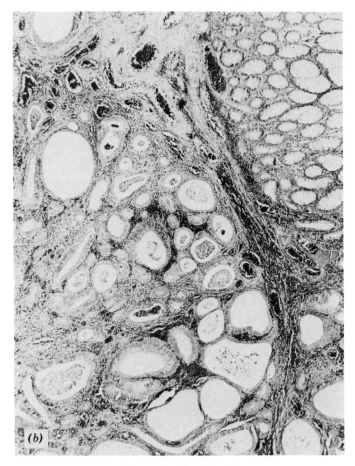

Figure 2. (*Continued*)

study. For instance, it has been estimated that an 8 to 10-cm margin in situ becomes about 4 to 5 cm when the tissue leaves the patient. Following formalin fixation, only 2 or 3 cm may remain as a margin (14).

In reporting the microscopic findings, the majority of tumors will be either grade II or III. Grade I tumors are generally small tumors associated with polyps (and really little different than those considered to be grade II). Grade IV tumors should have an additional description to indicate the distinctive features present, such as solid or anaplastic foci. Other features such as unusual inflammatory cell infiltrates and vascular permeation should also be mentioned. In addition to giving the Dukes classification, at Memorial Hospital we like to describe the depth of penetration quantitatively; for example, "extending superficially to muscularis propria," or "close to but not involving pericolic tissues," and so on. Occasionally, separate foci of the tumor are present in the pericolic fat, not recognizable as being in lymph nodes. These are described as such and considered as Dukes C lesions.

Adenocarcinoma

The common type of colonic adenocarcinoma is made up of uniform glandular structures, with mucin-containing epithelial elements. The differentiation is usually good or

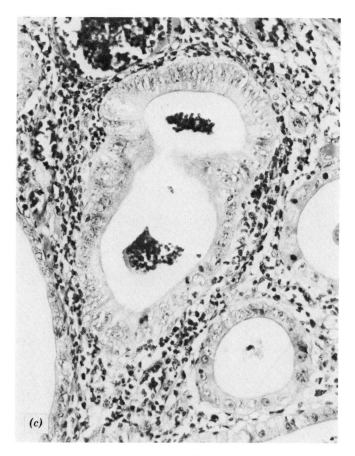

Figure 2. (*Continued*)

moderate. Poorly differentiated or anaplastic adenocarcinomas are rare, and, when diagnosed, the pathologist should reflect and be sure he or she is not dealing with a metastatic tumor, a melanoma, a carcinoid or a lymphoma.

Mucinous Adenocarcinoma

When a considerable proportion of an adenocarcinoma is mucin secreting, the designation mucinous is used. It is most often found in association with conventional adenocarcinoma in terms of histological appearance. A recent study has shown that tumors that were at least 60% mucin secreting in terms of pools of mucin with very little epithelium had a poorer prognosis than those with less mucin (15). The poor outlook was especially noteworthy when such tumors were located in the rectum.

Some cases of mucinous carcinoma may be difficult to diagnose. These are the rare instances of advanced colorectal cancers that appear as a fistulous tract, either in the anorectal region or as a rectovaginal fistula. Biopsies reveal pools of mucous and small amounts of purulent exudate. Cancer cells may be absent from the biopsy or so scant and inconspicuous as to be easily overlooked. Frequently, repeated biopsies are necessary before the true disease is uncovered. These cases have been described by Binkley and Quan (16) and Dukes and Galvin (17) (Fig. 4).

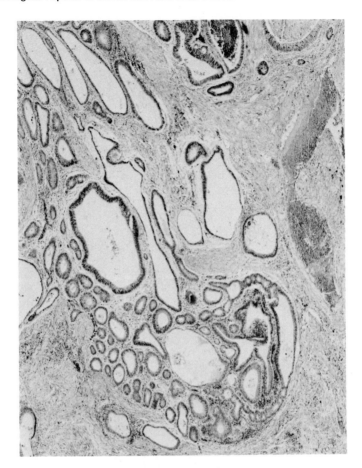

Figure 3. Another example of misplaced epithelium. This one shows dilated and cystic glands, a feature of some of these polyps and simulating colitis cystica profunda (9). An area such as this is less likely to be confused with carcinoma.

Signet-Ring Cell Adenocarcinoma

This adenocarcinoma resembles signet-ring carcinomas occurring elsewhere in the gastrointestinal tract, such as in the stomach. Indeed, one should be certain that a primary carcinoma elsewhere in the intestinal tract has been ruled out before considering such a tumor primary in the colon, rectum, or anus. They infiltrate diffusely and in situ changes are rarely found. In small biopsy specimens signet ring cells may be overshadowed by normal glandular elements (much in the manner of gastric signet-ring cancers) and the result may be an incorrect diagnosis. The cells may be diminutive, with barely any nuclear detail to evaluate, or they may be mistaken for histiocytes or other inflammatory cells. Omental biopsies of metastatic signet cell carcinoma, especially when sent as a frozen section, may be confused with inflammatory reactions, especially when desmoplasia is present. In rare instances, even when the presence of signet-ring cells is suspected, the diagnosis may have to await a mucin stain for confirmation.

Adenocarcinoma Arising in Ulcerative Colitis

One feature in particular about adenocarcinoma arising in ulcerative colitis deserves special mention. Many of these cancers are not exophytic in their growth pattern and tend to be flat, spreading laterally and deeply with little or insignificant luminal encroachment. For this reason, they can be difficult to detect by barium enema or by endoscopy (Fig. 5).

Metastases of Colon Carcinoma

Not infrequently, adenocarcinoma of the colon will metastasize to the ovary, vagina, or even to the vulva, where it may simulate a primary tumor. We have had submitted to us enlarged ovaries considered to be a primary ovarian neoplasm only to discover subsequently the origin to be a low rectal cancer. The lesion either was not seen with a barium enema or no barium enema was done. In one instance a vulvar metastasis was considered as a primary sweat gland adenocarcinoma; some months later the primary site was discovered in the colon.

These metastases resembled the primary colonic cancers, which were of the ordinary

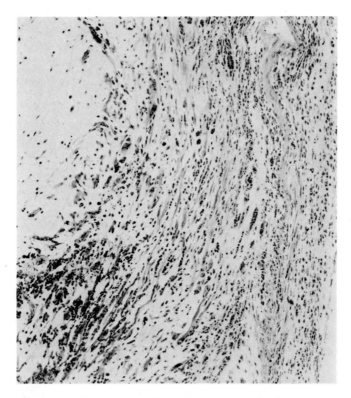

Figure 4. Purulent exudate with background of mucinous material in patient with an anal fistula. Several biopsies showed similar features and absence of tumor cells. Ultimately a resection revealed a typical mucinous adenocarcinoma as the basis for the fistulous tract, as well as the mucinous pools.

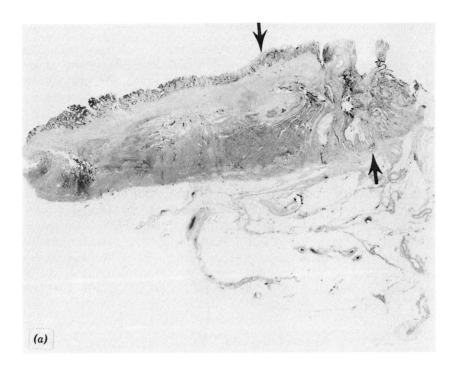

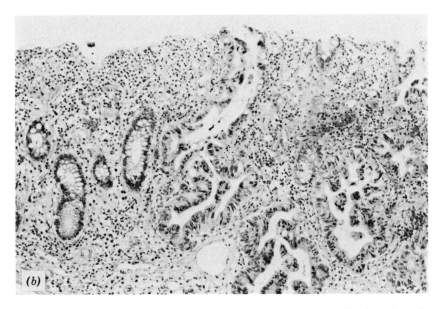

Figure 5. (*a*) Example of flat adenocarcinoma arising in a patient with ulcerative colitis. A stricture was suspected on the basis of barium enema findings; however, brushings obtained endoscopically revealed carcinoma and the colon was resected. The tumor extended into the pericolic fat and several lymph node metastases were found. (*b*) Atrophic mucosa with crypt loss, at left, and adenocarcinoma, at right [from area in (*a*) indicated by arrow in lumen]. (*c*) Infiltrating adenocarcinoma partially mucinous, extending to pericolic fat [from arrow located in mesocolon in (*a*)].

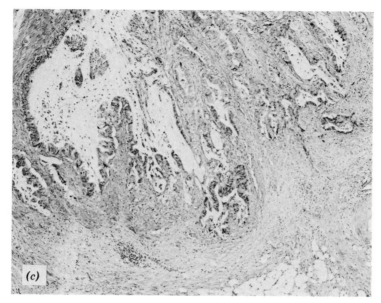

Figure 5. (*Continued*)

type. In the cases in which metastases were present in the ovary, the tumors did not look like the conventional papillary serous or mucinous carcinomas arising in the ovary. The vulvar and vaginal lesions also resembled the colonic primary. It was only because of the context of presentation and failure to consider another primary site that led to mistaken diagnoses at these sites (Fig. 6).

Prognostic Factors in Colon Cancer

A review by Zamcheck et al (18) revealed that such factors in colon cancer as the depth of bowel wall involvement (Dukes classification), grading of tumor (Broders method), cellular infiltrate (lymphocytic and plasma cell), vascular involvement (lymphatic, blood vessel), perineural invasion, and carcinoembryonic antigen (CEA) levels all had prognostic value.

Low serum levels of CEA suggested that the tumor was localized to the bowel wall. High levels indicated spread beyond the bowel. Lymphocyte and plasma cell infiltrate was found to confer a favorable prognosis (18,19). Tumors which were not well differentiated had a higher frequency of vascular and perineural involvement (20–22). These patients also had higher CEA levels.

SQUAMOUS CELL CARCINOMA OF COLON

Squamous carcinomas in the colon are rare. Most tumors of this type arise in the anorectal region. Less than 1% of all colon adenocarcinomas have squamous features (23). In rare instances a glandular component is absent and the tumor is entirely squamous. There is apparently a relatively higher incidence of adenosquamous carcinoma in patients with chronic ulcerative colitis [3 of 20 in the series reported by Comer et al

(24)]. In rare instances squamous metaplasia can be found in adenomatous polyps; this is a potential source of squamous carcinoma (Fig. 7).

LEIOMYOMA AND LEIOMYOSARCOMA

Smooth muscle tumors are rare in the large intestines as compared to other portions of the gastrointestinal tract. They are, however, more commonly found in the rectum than elsewhere in the large intestines. It has been estimated that about half the smooth muscle tumors of the colon and rectum are malignant; somewhat less than in the small intestines, where 80% are malignant (25).

Small tumors are occasionally discovered by palpation when within reach of the examining finger. Larger tumors, higher up, often are disclosed by bleeding after they have extended into and ulcerated through the mucosa. More often than not, pain is a significant symptom, especially with tumors arising in the rectum.

In general, the smaller tumors (less than 2 cm) are leiomyomas and larger tumors are sarcomatous, although there are notable exceptions. The benign tumors are orderly and have very few or no mitoses. Most leiomyosarcomas are obviously malignant in terms of

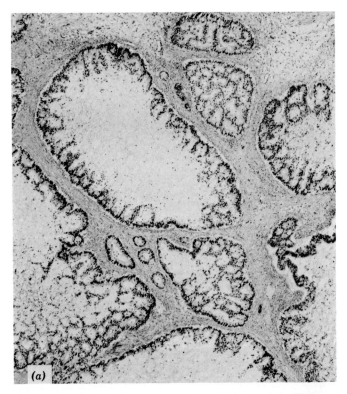

Figure 6. (*a*) Rectal adenocarcinoma metastatic to ovary. (*b*) Shows primary lesion in rectum. These tumors in the ovary are occasionally mistaken for a primary ovarian adenocarcinoma, especially when the colon cancer is occult.

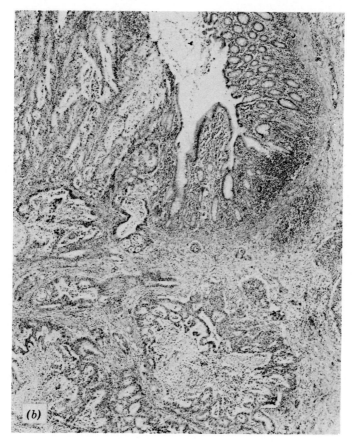

Figure 6. (*Continued*)

cellularity, nuclear and cellular variation in size and shape, and in mitotic activity. However, there remains a borderline group of lesions that appear banal and have very little mitotic activity but behave in a malignant fashion. Occasionally, recurrences or metastases are long-delayed. The diagnosis of a benign smooth muscle tumor should be made only when size and histology are carefully considered. Occasionally, leiomyosarcomas have long latent periods between the first operation and recurrence (26,27). Most, however, recur within a relative short time, varying from less than a year to several years (Figs. 8 and 9).

MALIGNANT MELANOMA OF THE ANUS AND RECTUM

Melanomas arise either in the anal skin or lower rectal tissues near the anorectal junction. The gross appearance can be deceptive, especially since many are nonpigmented. They appear as nodular growths and are often confused with thrombosed hemorrhoids or polyps. Fortunately, melanomas are quite rare in this location, in keeping with melanomas in general, which arise in or near mucous membranes. In one series (28), during a 29-year period, nine instances were encountered. This represented an incidence of

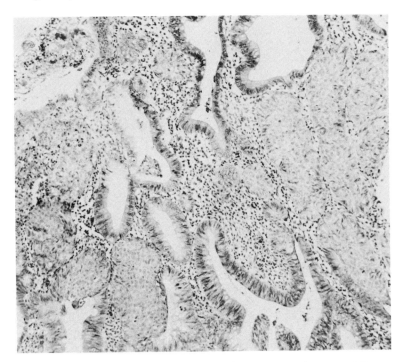

Figure 7. Solidly growing area in an adenomatous polyp resembling a uterine acanthoma. It is, perhaps, from such a focus that some epidermoid carcinomas arise in the large intestines.

0.25% of rectal adenocarcinomas, and 5 to 10% of the number of squamous carcinomas of the anus seen during the same period.

These cancers are, with few exceptions, fatal. Malignant malanomas of mucous membranes have always been recognized as having very poor prognosis, often attributed to an inherent virulence associated with those anatomic sites. It is more likely, however, that they are detected when they have reached a substantial size and, when compared to skin melanomas of similar size, are in fact no different in terms of behavior. Large melanomas which penetrate deeply and extend for relatively large distances into the underlying tissues have a very poor prognosis and this is precisely the case with anorectal melanomas.

The microscopic appearance is similar to melanomas arising in skin. There is a junctional component present, even when ulceration occurs, but many sections may be necessary to demonstrate it. Most anal melanomas are at least Clark level III or deeper, and more often than not the depth is measured in centimeters rather than millimeters or a fraction of a millimeter. Melanomas arising high up in rectal mucosa frequently have squamous metaplastic areas in which the tumor appears to arise; sometimes, however, the melanoma is present as such in the glandular epithelium (Fig. 10).

PERIANAL PAGET'S DISEASE AND BOWEN'S DISEASE

Paget's disease of the perianal skin can arise in several different ways. It may originate from a carcinoma arising in the adnexal skin structures, that is, as a sweat gland carcinoma, or it can develop from an adjoining mucinous carcinoma of the rectal tissues with secondary epidermal involvement. In a number of instances, the lesion appears confined to the epidermis with no apparent origin and no invasion. More often than not, however, repeated sectioning will reveal an associated sweat gland origin (29).

Microscopically, the type of Paget's disease that appears in the perianal skin is similar to that in the nipple and labia majora and vulvar regions. The tumor cells appear in the epithelium as either small nests or isolated cells, and the remaining epithelium appears normal. The type of Paget's disease that initially appears as isolated tumor cells in all layers of the epidermis is the kind most likely to be confused with Bowen's disease, which has the same type of pattern. The presence of mucin in the cytoplasm of the tumor cells will distinguish Paget's from Bowen's disease.

When the nesting of tumor cells occurs in the basal layers, the process may be confused with a primary melanoma. The distinction may be very difficult with

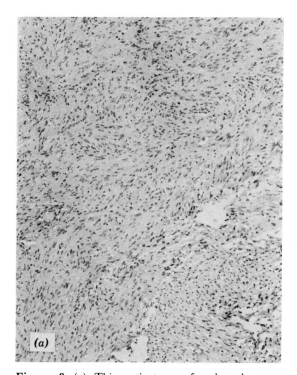

Figure 8. (*a*) This patient was found to have an adenocarcinoma of the sigmoid colon as well as a rectal mass. This frozen section biopsy of the rectal mass was considered to be a leiomyoma with atypia. (*b*) The paraffin section, which looked banal and not unlike a uterine leiomyoma, was diagnosed as benign. (*c*) The entire tumor was removed at a later date and revealed some portions which were considered to be leiomyosarcomatous. In this field there are several mitotic figures, but the cellular atypia is still not very marked (compare with Fig. 9). This patient, now 73 years old, has been free of recurrence for 7 years.

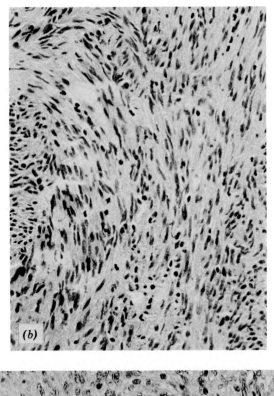

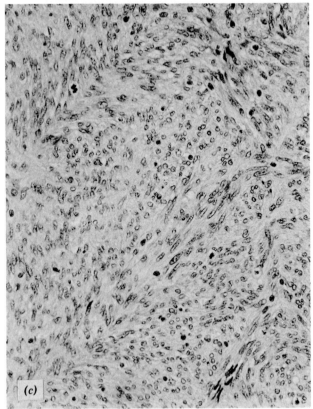

Figure 8. (*Continued*)

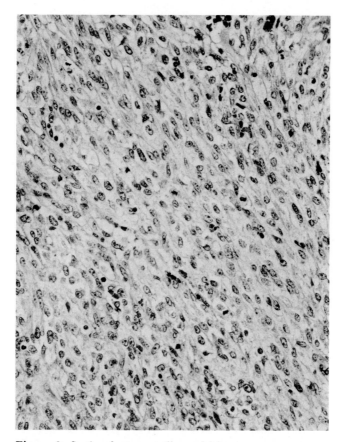

Figure 9. Section from a small rectal leiomyosarcoma measuring about 1 cm, removed by local excision in 1966. Shortly thereafter, an abdomino-perineal resection was performed and no residual tumor was present. Eleven years later, tumor was present in the pelvis and in the liver. This section is from the recurrence in the pelvis and shows a leiomyosarcoma with considerable atypia, cellularity, and many mitotic figures (compare with Fig. 8(c).

hematoxylin and eosin sections in some cases, but a mucin stain will reveal the difference (Fig. 11).

EPIDERMOID AND BASALOID CARCINOMAS OF THE ANUS AND ANAL CANAL

There are several types of carcinoma that can arise in the anal region. They have been variously called basaloid carcinoma, epidermoid carcinoma and transitional cloacogenic carcinoma. These are likely all variants of the same basic tumor. These tumors can arise from the anus, the anal canal, and at or above the pectinate line. They include a spectrum of histological features wherein they may be basaloid, that is, resembling transitional

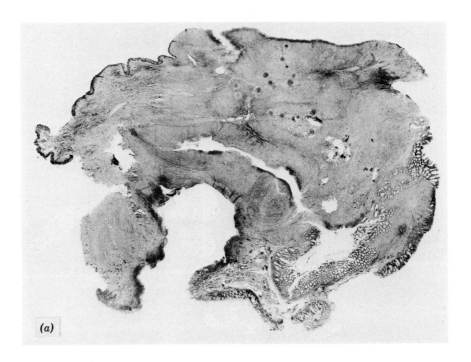

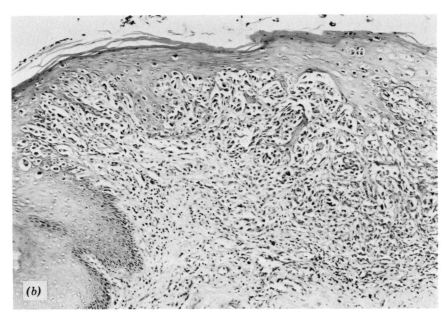

Figure 10. (*a*) This anorectal melanoma from a 71-year old man was 3 cm in diameter (3×). Metastases were present in 3 of 15 regional lymph nodes at the time of operation. The patient died 3 years later. (*b*) Junctional component is present in anal skin.

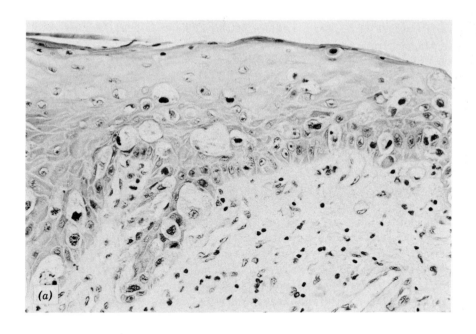

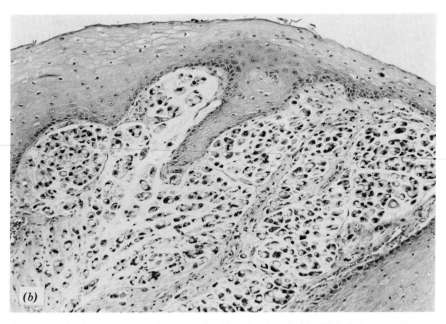

Figure 11. (*a*) Paget-type involvement of epidermis of anal skin. This lesion actually came from a signet-ring cell carcinoma located higher up in the rectum. (*b*) In other portions of the anal skin the typical signet-ring cells are present.

cell carcinomas of the bladder, squamous and keratinizing, or both. Most tumors have a combination of features; a number are almost all "basaloid," others have only a few squamous foci, and still others are mainly keratinizing.

Variations of these histological features have been used in classifying such tumors in an attempt to determine prognosis. This has been difficult and conflicting reports have resulted. The problem is that each type of predominant microscopic pattern must be matched properly with the other types. In other words, the tumors in one group must be matched with tumors in another so that both groups have an equal number of cases wherein the tumor is about the same size, is at the same location and the same clinical stage when first observed, and is then treated in a like manner. In the absence of such matched "controls," little can be said of prognosis of the different types.

Some studies have indicated that the so-called histologically pure basaloid tumor (about one-fifth of all anal cancers) is probably a relatively low-grade tumor in terms of size when discovered and is less likely to metastasize. Patients who have tumors with anaplastic foci (epidermoid with nuclear anaplasia), which are thus of a higher grade, have a poorer prognosis (30). In other studies, patients with tumors of less than 2 cm did best, while those with larger tumors showed significant falloff in cures. Other studies also showed that high-grade tumor patients did less well, as would be expected (31).

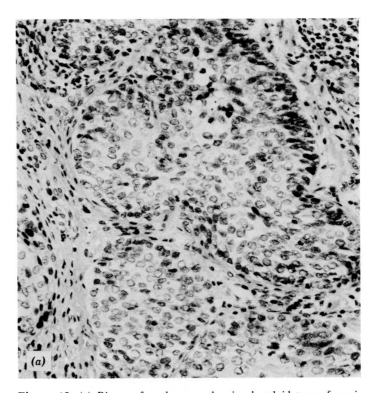

Figure 12. (*a*) Biopsy of anal tumor showing basaloid type of carcinoma. (*b*) One year later, following chemotherapy and radiation therapy, a recurrence was noted and biopsied. The lesion showed epidermoid features with keratinization, probably a spontaneous change, but an effect of therapy cannot be excluded.

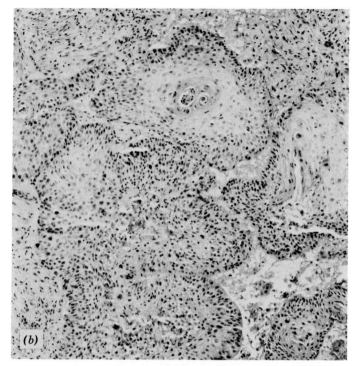

Figure 12. (*Continued*)

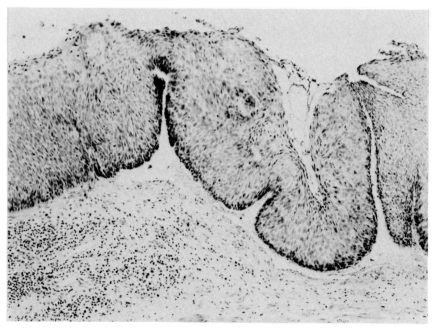

Figure 13. In situ changes in an anal carcinoma. In this instance, even the noninfiltrating lesion had a basaloid appearance.

These epidermoid and basaloid tumors comprise about 2 to 3% of all cancers in this region. A rarer type of anorectal cancer is the mucoepidermoid carcinoma. About one of these is seen for every 12 ordinary carcinomas in this region (32). Mucoepidermoid carcinomas generally are easily recognized and their mucous features are noticeable even without a specific stain. The prognosis is a 5-year survival rate of 57%, similar to that of the low-grade basaloid anal cancers (Figs. 12 and 13).

CARCINOID TUMORS

Carcinoid tumors occur more often in the small intestines and appendix than in the large intestines. These tumors have been discovered in all parts of the colon, but about one-third are found in the cecum; the remainder are distributed more or less equally in the ascending, transverse, and sigmoid colon (33). In addition to the cecum, the rectum is another site of predilection for these tumors (34).

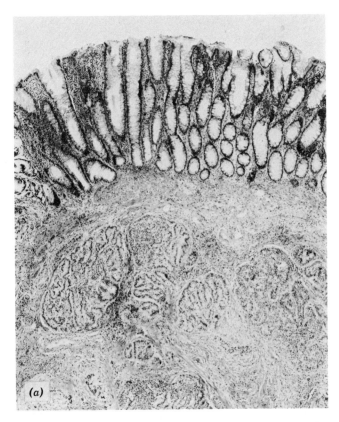

Figure 14. (a) Rectal carcinoid in submucosa with intact overlying mucosa. (b) This pattern with glandular features can be confused with a conventional rectal adenocarcinoma. The Grimelius stain (36) in this instance was positive, an unusual feature in a rectal carcinoid. The mucin stain was negative.

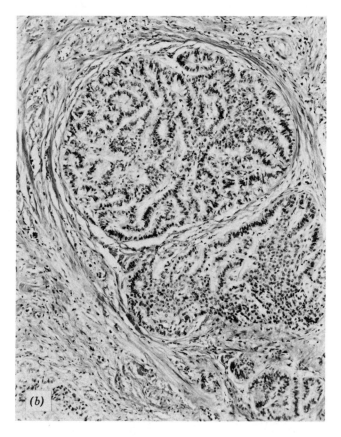

Figure 14. (*Continued*)

Those in the colon are often quite large, averaging close to 5 cm, with a diameter of 0.5 to 15 cm in one series (33). Metastases are found more frequently in colonic carcinoids than those arising elsewhere. Medium-sized tumors (4.7 cm) did not metastasize, but tumors 6.1 cm in size did (33).

Rectal carcinoids are much smaller when discovered than those found in the colon. In the series reported by Quan, et al (34), there were 33 tumors less than 1 cm; 9 tumors were between 1 and 2 cm and 4 patients had tumors greater than 2 cm. Those tumors larger than 2 cm were malignant; one that was smaller than 2 cm was also malignant. All the large ones had nodal or liver metastases. (The one small carcinoid recurred as a pararectal mass 5 years after primary excision and was free from recurrence at least 7 years thereafter.)

The histologic pattern of the colonic carcinoids may have a rosette or pseudoglandular pattern (type C) or solid nests, sometimes with desmoplasia to form cords or trabeculae (type A) or both patterns (35). The rectal carcinoids may also have a type A pattern with desmoplasia as well as a ribbon pattern (type B) (35). The carcinoid tumors that have one of the classical patterns are generally not difficult to diagnose. Occasionally, when the glandular or adenomatous pattern is prominent, such tumors may be mistaken for ordinary colonic adenocarcinomas. The diagnostic problems arise when a small

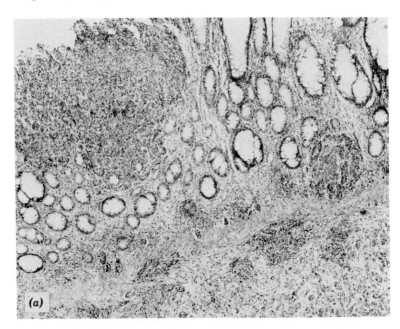

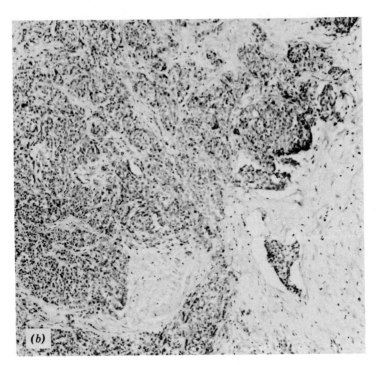

Figure 15. (*a*) Diffusely infiltrating "small cell" tumor of rectum, considered to be a carcinoid because of trabecular pattern and small cellular nests. The Grimelius stain was negative, but mucin was present in the cytoplasm of many of these small cells. (*b*) Tumor involves mucosa and muscularis propria with lymphatic invasion.

biopsy, often crushed, contains a few solid nests of dark staining cells; these may be m
taken for lymphomas or considered "anaplastic carcinomas." Sometimes, especially with
an intact and normal mucosa, a few carcinoid nests in the submucosa may be easily
overlooked. The diagnosis, however, depends on the morphologic traits as disclosed by
conventional stains. Colon and rectal carcinoids with rare exceptions are not argyro-
philic and they do not take the argentaffin stain.

The carcinoid syndrome is rare in patients with carcinoid tumors of the colon (33).
No case of carcinoid syndrome arising from a rectal carcinoid has been noted (Figs. 14
and 15).

ACKNOWLEDGEMENTS

The assistance of Martha Klapp in the preparation of this chapter is gratefully
acknowledged. The excellent photographs were prepared by Margaret Uibel and
Pamela Post.

REFERENCES

1. Muto T, Bussey HJR, Morson BC: The evolution of cancer of the colon and rectum. *Cancer* 36:2251, 1975.

2. Quan SHQ, Castro EB: Papillary adenomas (villous tumors): A review of 215 cases. *Dis Colon Rectum* 14:267, 1971.

3. Fenoglio CM, Kaye GI, Lane N: Distribution of human colonic lymphatics in normal, hyperplastic, and adenomatous tissue. *Gastroenterol* 64:51, 1973.

4. Morson BC, Bussey HJR: Predisposing Causes of Intestinal Cancer. *Current Problems in Surgery.* Chicago, Year Book Medical Publishers, 1970.

5. Shatney CH, Lober PH, Gilbertson V, et al: Management of focally malignant pedunculated adenomatous colorectal polyps. *Dis Colon Rectum* 19:334, 1976.

6. Lane N, Kay GI: Pedunculated adenomatous polyp of the colon with carcinoma, lymph node metastasis, and suture-line recurrence. *Am J Clin Pathol* 48:170, 1976.

7. Muto T, Bussey HJR, Morson BC: Pseudo-carcinomatous invasion in adenomatous polyps of the colon and rectum. *J Clin Path* 26:25, 1973.

8. Greene FL: Epithelial misplacement in adenomatous polyps of the colon and rectum. *Cancer* 33:206, 1974.

9. Fechner RE: Polyp of the colon possessing features of colitis cystica profunda. *Dis Colon Rectum* 10:359, 1967.

10. Collins JO, Falk M, Guibone R: Benign lymphoid polyposis of the colon: a case report. *Pediatrics* 38:897, 1966.

11. Wolfson JJ, Goldstein G, Krivit W, et al. Lymphoid hyperplasia of the large intestine associated with dysgammaglobulinemia. *Am J Roentgenol* 108:610, 1970.

12. Theander G, Trágårdh B: Lymphoid hyperplasia of the colon in childhood. *Acta Radiol (Diagn) Fasc 5,* 17:631, 1976.

13. Edelman MJ, Sternberg SS: Nodular lymphoid hyperplasia of the colon in an adult. *Clin Bull* 7:146, 1977.

14. Dunphy JE, Broderick EG: A critique of anterior resection in the treatment of cancer of the rectum and pelvic colon. *Surgery* 30:106, 1951.

15. Symonds DA, Vickery AL Jr: Mucinous carcinoma of the colon and rectum. *Cancer* 37:1891, 1976.

16. Binkley GE, Quan SHQ: Pseudoinflammatory colloid carcinoma of the rectum. *Cancer* 7:1020, 1954.

17. Dukes CE, Galvin C: Colloid carcinoma arising within fistulae in the ano-rectal region. *Ann Roy Coll Surg Engl* 18:246, 1956.

18. Zamcheck N, Doos WG, Prudente R, et al: Prognostic factors in colon carcinoma. Correlation of serum carcinoembryonic antigen level and tumor histopathology. *Human Path.* 6:31, 1975.

19. Spratt JS, Spjut HJ: Prevalence and prognosis of individual clinical and pathological variables associated with colorectal carcinoma. *Cancer* 20:1976, 1967.

20. Grinnell RS: The grading and prognosis of carcinoma of the colon and rectum. *Ann Surg* 109:500, 1939.

21. Seefield PH, Bargen JA: The spread of carcinoma of the rectum: invasion of lymphatics, veins and nerves. *Ann Surg* 118:76, 1943.

22. Sunderland DA: The significance of vein invasion by cancer of the rectum and sigmoid. *Cancer* 2:429, 1949.

23. Crissman JD: Adenosquamous and squamous cell carcinoma of the colon. *Am J Surg Path* 2:47, 1978.

24. Comer TP, Beahrs OH, Dockerty MB: Primary squamous cell carcinoma and adenoacanthoma of the colon. *Cancer* 28:1111, 1971.

25. Anderson PA, Dockerty MB, Buie LA: Myomatous tumors of the rectum (leiomyomas and myosarcomas). *Surgery* 28:642, 1950.

26. Quan SHQ, Berg JW: Leiomyoma and leiomyosarcoma of the rectum. *Dis Colon Rectum* 5:415, 1962.

27. Matsuda T, Condon RE: Leiomyosarcoma of the colon with metastasis to the liver: right hepatic lobectomy in presence of variant hepatic artery. *J Surg Oncol* 3:533, 1971.

28. Morson BC: Rare malignant tumours of the rectum and anal region, in Dukes, CE (ed): *Cancer of the Rectum.* Edinburgh and London, E & S Livingston, Ltd, 1960, chap. VIII, p. 80.

29. Williams SL, Rogers LW, Quan SHQ: Perianal Paget's disease. Report of seven cases. *Dis Colon Rectum* 19:30, 1976.

30. Lone F, Berg JW, Stearns MW Jr: Basaloid tumors of the anus. *Cancer* 13:907, 1960.

31. Klotz RG Jr, Pamukcoglu T, Souilliard DH: Transitional cloacogenic carcinoma of the anal canal. Clinicopathologic study of three hundred seventy five cases. *Cancer* 20:1727, 1967.

32. Berg JW, Lone F, Stearns MW Jr: Mucoepidermoid anal cancer. *Cancer* 13:914, 1960.

33. Berardi RS: Carcinoid tumors of the colon (exclusive of the rectum): Review of the literature. *Dis Colon Rectum* 15:383, 1972.

34. Quan SHQ, Bader G, Berg JW: Carcinoid tumors of the rectum. *Dis Colon Rectum* 7:197, 1964.

35. Dawson IMP: The endocrine cells of the gastrointestinal tract and the neoplasms which arise from them, in Morson, BC (ed): *Pathology of the Gastro-Intestinal Tract.* Berlin, Heidelberg, New York, Springer-Verlag, 1976, p. 221.

36. Lack EE, and Mercer L: A modified Grimelius argyrophil technique for neurosecretory granules. *Am J Surg Path* 1:275, 1977.

5

The Management of Adenomas of the Large Gut

Ralph E. L. Hertz

INTRODUCTION

General Principles

The risk of cancer at the time of excision or as a subsequent development is the overriding consideration in the surgery of adenomas of the large gut. The surgeon should, therefore, always plan total excision of the lesion or lesions with preservation of an intact specimen suitable for evaluation by the pathologist, who must be able to determine if removal is complete and to detect and properly stage areas of malignant change within the lesion. The excision of adenomas in fragments is to be avoided whenever possible. The surgeon must bear in mind the tendency to multiplicity of adenomas and the increased likelihood of coexisting adenocarcinomas. Diagnostic and therapeutic measures should allow for these facts. The operative procedures used to accomplish these objectives vary from simple total biopsy or cautery snare excision to total coloproctectomy.

The method of choice for the removal of adnomas is determined by their size, shape, number, and location. Adenomas are generally considered pedunculated or sessile, but every conceivable combination of these forms is encountered in individual or coexistent lesions. The pedunculated form usually consists of a bulbous head, which is the adenoma, and a pedicle, formed by traction, which is covered with normal mucosa. In some instances the adenoma covers the entire pedicle and extends to the plane of the bowel wall. In others an apparently pedunculated lesion is, in fact, a traction protrusion from a sessile adenoma which may extend over several centimeters. The sessile portion may be elevated only 2 to 3 mm and, therefore, may be difficult to delineate from the adjacent normal mucosa.

All adenomas should be removed regardless of the degree of difficulty as they are precursor lesions to invasive cancer. This statement must be tempered with judgment, particularly as relates to the elderly or poor risk patient, since growth and transitional changes in adenomas may occur over a period of many years. Furthermore, malignancy at any stage is unusual in adenomas under 1 cm in size. On the other hand, the clinician must appreciate that the assumption that a given lesion is an adenoma rather than a carcinoma is, at best, an educated guess with a significant incidence of error. This is particularly true of the problem case where the advisability of surgery is under question due to the combination of significant size and relative inaccessibility of the lesion. The rate of growth shown by barium enema is not reliable evidence of the benign or malignant state of a supposed adenoma, based on the thesis that a slow increment indicates the benign state. An adenoma may be almost totally replaced by adenocarcinoma and may even exhibit regional node metastasis without significant recent size increment (1–4).

The Physical Characteristics of Adenomas

The physical forms of adenomas as well as their histologic characteristics fuse into one another so that many variants occur. Nevertheless, in the discussion of management it is best to consider adenomas separately as pedunculated and sessile forms. The histologic pattern has essentially no bearing on management.

The intestinal adenoma is a unique lesion in that it arises from a simple mucosal layer which is separated from adjacent deep structures by distinct mobile layers. These growths occur within a muscular tube and are subjected to traction by peristaltic action. It is through this mechanism that a pedicle is formed, the adenoma drawing with it the mobile mucosa and superficial layers of the submucosa, but not its deep layers or the muscularis propria. The resultant lesion can be excised at the base of the pedicle without perforation of the bowel wall, providing that a low-level current is used with resultant minimal adjacent wall necrosis. Similarly, when traction is applied to a sessile lesion it tends to elevate at a plane between the mucosa and the deep layers of the submucosa, thus minimizing the risk of perforation. This is in distinct contrast to other lesions that arise within the layers of the bowel wall. For instance, an apparently pedunculated lipoma of the large gut may contain the muscularis propria and the peritoneum at the summit of the pedicle.

In the case of the pedunculated adenoma the tumor is widely separated from the deep layers of the bowel wall. When cancer develops in such a lesion, invasion to the level of the muscularis propria is a late phenomenon. These adenomas lend themselves to easy excision and provide specimens with a relatively small distinct area for the pathologist to study the interface between tumor and normal structures. On the other hand, large sessile lesions may present difficult problems in excision. The tumor lies close to the deep layers of the bowel wall, so that cancer arising within it has a greater potential for invasion of these structures. Accurate evaluation by the pathologist may be exceedingly difficult due to the size of the tumor, the extent of the interface, and the limitations of the material presented to him. The differing nature of these problems is highlighted in Figure 1. Here certain effects of pedunculation upon a lesion are compared to a sessile lesion of similar surface dimension. The separation of invasive cancer developing within the pedunculated lesion from the deep structues of the wall is apparent. The interface for surgical transection and pathologic study in the former is approximately 1% of the latter. The management of the sessile form is obviously much more difficult, although the basic pathologic process is the same.

Role of Biopsy

Partial biopsy has a limited application in the management of adenomas of the large gut. Adenomas commonly show great variation of histologic pattern within a single

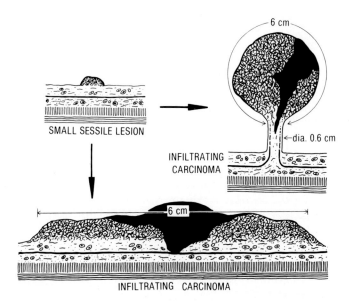

SMALL SESSILE LESION

INFILTRATING CARCINOMA

←dia. 0.6 cm

6 cm

6 cm

INFILTRATING CARCINOMA

Figure 1. As a small sessile lesion grows it may either become pedunculated or remain sessile. Adenomas of these respective configurations with comparable dimensions and containing infiltrating cancer (denoted in solid black) within them are shown. The interface between tumor and normal structures at the level of the pedicle is 3.1416×0.3 cm^2 or 0.28 cm^2, whereas that in the sessile lesion is 3.1416×3 cm^2 or 28.27 cm^2, a hundredfold increase.

lesion, from the benign state to invasive cancer, so that evaluation must depend upon as complete an assessment as feasible. The tissue sample of a partial biopsy is small, may not be representative of the entire lesion, and cannot be properly oriented. The information thus obtained is inconclusive and may be misleading. Biopsy is principally used, but only infrequently indicated, for the confirmation of the clinician's impression that a sessile lesion is benign. Information thus obtained must be carefully applied. The intact excised lesion is the proper biopsy specimen.

Instruments

There are instruments which have been specifically designed for the treatment of lesions of the anus, rectum, and colon. Others have a more general application but enhance treatment capability in this area. There are certain features of these instruments which we at MSKCC have found to be important.

High-Intensity Headlights

These units greatly facilitate work through anoscopes and through proctoscopes of 2.5-cm diameter and greater. They are indispensable for many direct transanal excisions. There are three types of suitable lights: the halogen beam, the large bundle fiber optic, and selected high-intensity incandescent units. The first type has the disadvantage of excessive heat production during lengthy procedures.

Proctoscopes, Sigmoidoscopes,
and Rigid Colonoscopes

These instruments should be equipped with a distal light so that intraluminal instruments will not interfere with illumination. A fiber-optic source is ideal because of its trouble-free operation and lack of heat production. The light carrier should be retractable for at least a few centimeters with maintenance of adequate field illumination so that work can be continued when a pedunculated lesion or other material enters the end of the instrument. It should be readily removable for cleansing. The carrier is best placed in a small channel on the outside of the instrument.

The most suitable proctoscope or sigmoidoscope for management of a specific case is the shortest and widest that can be passed without undue difficulty to the necessary level; such an instrument provides maximum visualization and control. On the other hand, the smaller-diameter instruments can be passed to higher levels in a much greater proportion of cases, and they cause less patient discomfort. It is obvious that any size increment in the diameter of the instrument must be multiplied by a factor of 3.14 in terms of the resultant increased stretching of the bowel. The surgeon should have a wide variety of these instruments available, in lengths from 10 to 50 cm, with an outside diameter (OD) of 1.1 to 3.5 cm. The larger calibers, that is, above 2.5 cm OD, are useful only for proctoscopes and short sigmoidoscopes. The high-intensity headlight provides excellent illumination for these large-caliber instruments. We most often use instruments of 1.7 cm OD or larger for excisional work, but with proper instrumentation this can be accomplished for a wide variety of lesions through the 1.3 cm OD instrument. The 1.1-cm-OD instrument is quite adequate for examination and biopsy. The maximum degree of interchangeability of components within the system should be achieved, so that the widest range of instrumentation is available for the lowest initial cost and maintenance. Instruments of this type are shown in Figure 2.

The Cautery Snare

The cautery-snare instrument should minimize visual interference at the handle level and should be equipped with as thin a cannula or carrier as possible while still providing reasonable stability and good insulating capacity. There should be minimal resistance to movement of the snare to preserve a fine sense of touch. The potential range of motion in the handle should be no less than 6 cm to permit the use of large loops when necessary. Fine, monofilament, nonrigid snare wires with some spring and yet with a degree of malleability is essential to achieve the maximum potential of the method. We have found spring wire of 0.005 through 0.010 in. diameter to be suitable, but various alloys and commercially available snares may be used. The use of a fine copper rod carrier with soldered snare loops permits individual loop selection and formation appropriate to the lesion to be excised. The cannula and carriers should be available in varied working lengths for operation through the full range of rigid endoscopes to the 50-cm length. These simple instruments allow excision of most lesions located from the anus to the upper sigmoid, and frequently to a location as high as the splenic flexure.

There is a vast array of power sources with differing current-output characteristics available for use with the cautery snare. We have found a low-level coagulating current to be most effective. The current should exhibit frequent peaks to offer sufficient hemostasis. The unit should be designed to minimize variations in output with changes in the operative field. No specific power output setting can be recommended, since the setting will vary with the unit and with the instrumentation, including the wire gauge

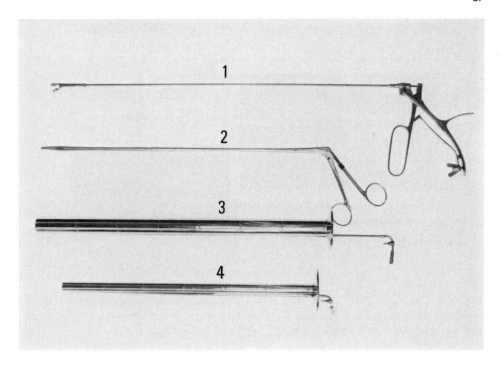

Figure 2. (*1*) Biopsy or excisional cup with universal handle. (*2*) Alligator or pickup forceps, noncutting. (*3*) 35-cm (2.0 cm o.d.) operating sigmoidoscope with light carrier retracted 5 cm. (*4*) 30-cm (1.3 cm o.d.) sigmoidoscope; excellent for routine sigmoidoscopy and a useful operative caliber.

used. It is a good practice to check the coagulating effect of the loop at the planned setting on adjacent normal mucosa routinely before becoming committed to a specific excision. The snare loop is then carefully placed and approximated to the tissue to be transected. A low-level current is then applied briefly without movement of the loop, following which the loop is slowly closed with constant current application. The output may be increased if necessary during the transection, and a low-level blended cutting current may be added if undue tissue resistance is encountered. The surgeon should become familiar with the performance characteristics of one unit and then should attempt to use it whenever possible. A suitable type of cautery-snare handle and carrier and snare loops is shown in Figure 3.

Biopsy Cup
The traditional heavy-box type of so-called proctologic biopsy instrument should never be used. An excellent biopsy instrument is the small cup, which is used with a universal handle and a cannula of any desired length. Two to four sizes of biopsy cup, varying from 4 to 9 mm in diameter, should be available for the appropriate biopsy or excision.

Alligator or Pick-Up Forceps
These noncutting forceps serve to pick up specimens, to apply material for hemostasis or cleansing, or as hemostats to which a coagulating current can be applied. The forceps must have a reasonably long jaw and be of adequately rigid design and long enough to

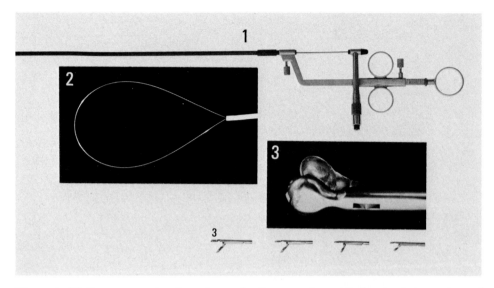

Figure 3. (*1*) Cautery snare handle and cannula. Constructed to minimize visual obstruction and resistance. (*2*) Cautery snare loop. Malleable and of varied gauge and dimension. (*3*) Biopsy cups. Varied dimensions: 9 mm, 7 mm, 5 mm, and 3 mm, and detail of cup.

function through the longest sigmoidoscope to be used. A forceps of this type of suitable length should be available whenever transsigmoidoscopic excision is to be performed.

Flexible Fiber-Optic Colonoscope

Flexible colonoscopes provide directional control of the tip and are constructed with multiple channels for instrumentation, cleansing of the field, and insufflation. Flexible fiber-optic colonoscopes have greatly increased the incidence of successful transanal examination and excision of lesions proximal to the upper sigmoid, and they have made the examination of the area proximal to the splenic flexure possible for the first time. The entire colon can be visualized in approximately 90% of cases. There is an abundant current literature describing these instruments, and design development is progressing so rapidly that they will not be described in detail here.

SESSILE ADENOMAS

The term sessile adenoma has often been mistakenly equated with the villous adenoma, which in turn has been considered synonymous with the papillary adenoma. Sessile adenomas of all histologic variants occur and range in size from less than 1 cm^2 to annular lesions covering over 100 cm^2. The terms villous adenoma or villous tumor should be restricted to the description of a clinical entity that consists of a large sessile lesion with a soft frondlike surface which exudes abundant mucous. Such a lesion characteristically has poorly defined margins that fuse almost imperceptibly with the adjacent mucosa. It is best to restrict this term to lesions that essentially fulfill these criteria and are 3 cm or greater in diameter. These lesions are predominantly of the papillary type. They carry a high risk of malignant change. They are occasionally associated with severe hypokalemia due to an abundant mucous secretion with high potassium loss.

Villous tumors, particularly of the rectum, historically are known to have a high incidence of postexcision local recurrence. This has not been our experience when an apparently adequate excision has been performed. We have seen a few instances of limited local recurrence among large lesions under these circumstances, but the recurrences have subsequently been controlled by simple local excision. The problem of repeated significant local recurrence has been limited to cases where the adequacy of excision has been compromised because of high operative risk, advanced age of the patient, or reluctance to carry out an abdominoperineal resection. We have not lost any patients to invasive cancer among these recurrent cases (5).

General Principles

There are certain principles which should be followed in the treatment of sessile adenomas: (*1*) As careful a determination as possible must be made that the lesion is benign and it should then be treated as such. (*2*) Preexcisional biopsy is generally not indicated, and if it is performed, it is primarily to confirm a clinical impression and not to form it. It must be interpreted with caution. If such a biopsy is done, this should be by the responsible surgeon as prior biopsy is often difficult to interpret, and the resultant induration interferes with evaluation of the lesion. (*3*) If there is doubt whether a lesion should be considered benign or malignant it is usually best to carry out local total excision when this is feasible, and then return for a proper cancer operation if indicated. (*4*) Procedures that entail entering the mesentery and lymphatic drainage area of the tumor should be avoided whenever possible. If segmental resection is necessary it should include an adequate mesenteric resection. (*5*) If transabdominal excision is performed, the entire colonic mucosa should be cleared of further mucosal lesions by measures beyond that of the barium enema; that is, by preoperative flexible colonoscopy or intraoperative colotomy and coloscopy; unsuspected lesions are discovered in about half the cases using these procedures.

Treatment

The important considerations in selecting procedures for the removal of sessile adenomas are the location and size of the lesion. For the purpose of discussing appropriate techniques, the rectum and the colon can be divided into three segments: the low and mid-rectum, the upper rectum, and the colon. The tumors are frequently of such large dimensions that they involve more than one of these segments. There are few other instances where such careful judgment is required in the selection of the appropriate surgical procedure, because of the combination of difficult anatomic features, the problem of a lesion that can range from benign to fully malignant, and the frequent complications of advanced age and poor surgical risk.

Small sessile lesions up to 1 cm in diameter are best removed by biopsy cup excision whenever feasible, since this procedure supplies the optimum pathologic specimen. Bleeding from the base is easily controlled by simple pressure, the application of Gelfoam, or coagulation.

Cautery-snare excision is appropriate at all levels, either through rigid or flexible instruments, provided the lesion is excised as a single specimen or at most as a definite total excision in two cuts. The extent to which cautery-snare excision can be utilized will depend upon the experience of the operator. As a general statement, larger lesions can be removed with greater safety in the extraperitoneal rectum, and both size restriction and hazard of perforation increase at intraperitoneal levels.

Low and Midrectum

A wide variety of methods are available to cope with the many problems of this area. The cautery-snare technique is applicable even to large lesions with the use of specially formed loops of appropriate gauge, since excellent exposure and control can be obtained with the use of large-caliber operating proctoscopes or retractors. Furthermore, since much of the segment is extraperitoneal the risk of perforation and serious complication is minimal.

Direct transanal excision is applicable to most lesions except the largest. The addition of posterior sphincterotomy does help the exposure but is rarely required unless restrictive abnormalities of the anal canal are present. The smaller lesions can be excised with traction applied by a noncrushing clamp such as a Babcock clamp, or by a few superficial mattress sutures placed distinctly beyond the margins of the tumor. The larger lesions are best removed by the double-row traction suture technique described below. The following requirements must be met to take advantage the full potential of the method. Illumination should be excellent and may be achieved with a high-intensity headlight. Exposure must be adequate; a self-retaining anal retractor such as the Parks instrument is suitable for small-to-moderate-sized lesions, but exposure of the larger ones can only be obtained by firm traction serially directed in the axis of the work. The operating instruments must be of sufficient length and rigidity but of minimal bulk. the last requirement, but not the least, is that skilled assistance is mandatory.

A wide range of sessile adenomas can effectively be excised by the technique shown in Figure 4, the essential feature of which is the placement of a double row of marking-traction mattress sutures distinctly beyond the circumference of the tumor. The first row of sutures is laid approximately 5 mm beyond the visible margins of the lesion and the second at approximately 7 mm beyond the first. These sutures are left long and the rows are held by distinctly different clamps. The sutures are applied starting distally and advancing proximally; thus, the lower ones can be used for traction to displace the upper portions of the lesion caudad for progressive application. The sutures should be placed deeply enough to include the submucosa and preferably even the superficial fibers of the muscularis propria. In this manner the surgeon is assured of a distinct peripheral line for the excision of the lesion even if the field is temporarily covered by blood or mucous.

The periphery of the incision should be developed close to the outside row of sutures, and the depth of the plane of excision must be at least against the muscularis propria. There is considerable advantage to including a thin layer of muscularis propria in the excision, especially under any areas of undue induration. This procedure has not produced complications and offers the most meaningful specimens for pathological evaluation. A solution of epinephrine may be infiltrated into the submucosal layer to reduce bleeding, but in most cases this should not be necessary. The excision base is left open, although it may be reduced somewhat in size by the tying together of selected sutures of the outer rim. In spite of the extent of the denuded area, bleeding is controlled without undue difficulty and delayed bleeding is rare. Major complications of this technique are virtually nonexistent. Postoperative stricturing does not occur.

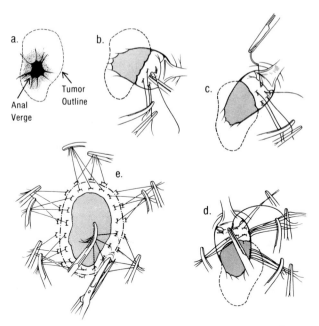

Figure 4. (*a*) Outline of sessile tumor projected through perianal area. (*b–d*) Progressive placement of tagged double row of mattress sutures around tumor, with firm retraction in axis of work. (*e*) Excision of tumor is commenced caudad with incision line close to outer suture row.

Posterior proctotomy with coccygectomy, to which may be added excision of the lower one or two segments of the sacrum if necessary, is an excellent technique. It provides wide access to the rectum, which may be entered near the midline or may be rotated as needed. Excision of the lesion is carried out at the plane described for the transanal approach, although full-thickness excision is readily done if indicated. However, this approach transgresses the lymphatic drainage area of the tumor, and it may compromise later, more radical surgery. It also carries an inherent risk of fistula formation, although the risk is minimal. The method should be employed only when transanal excision is not practicable because of a combination of limitation of access at the anorectum and the size and location of the tumor. Access at the anorectum may be restricted either by specific pathology or by physical features such as a combination of a high levator shelf and a restricted bony inlet.

There are instances when, due to size, high location, and/or extensive spread to the crypt level, these lesions are unsuited for the local procedures previously described. The lesions must then be managed by anterior resection, a pullthrough procedure or even abdomino-perineal resection with permanent colostomy. These procedures are undertaken for what is considered benign disease, so the dissection is performed immediately deep to the plane of the mesentery in the upper pelvis and approximately halfway to the pelvic walls in the low pelvis, relating to the middle and inferior hemorrhoidal distribution. The dissection provides less than the maximum lymphatic excision desirable for infiltrating cancer, but it minimizes the risk of bladder or sexual dysfunction as well as that of anastomotic leakage in those cases suitable for anterior resection.

Upper Rectum

Many cases involving this area are suitable for cautery-snare excision. Transanal excision can be utilized in some instances as the mobility of the area may permit downward displacement by traction. Posterior proctotomy with coccygectomy is almost never applicable. A transabdominal approach is frequently indicated and can be carried out by either of two methods. If prior proctoscopy and transabdominal palpation both indicate that simple excision is adequate proctotomy through the serosal aspect of the bowel provides ready access. On the other hand, if segmental resection is deemed necessary a margin of at least three centimeters should be obtained distal to the lesion and twelve centimeters or more proximally. The mesenteric resection should be full thickness, corresponding to the resection line distally, and carried cephalad to the origin of the left colic artery.

Colon

Most of the smaller sessile lesions of the colon can be excised by the cautery-snare technique, using either rigid instruments or via the flexible colonoscope. It is best to limit this approach to lesions 2 cm or less, because of the risk of perforation and/or incomplete excision in dealing with larger lesions.

The larger lesions must be excised by a transabdominal approach and the method of choice is dependent upon the specifics of the case, including the characteristics of the lesion or lesions, and the age and operative risk of the patient. A solitary, typically benign lesion is best managed by the procedure of simple colotomy and local excision, which carries the lowest possible chance of operative morbidity and mortality. The surgeon will only rarely have to recommend subsequent additional surgery based upon the discovery of significant infiltrating cancer in the lesion. On the other hand, if resection is deemed necessary for the initial management of the lesion, the procedure should then include an appropriate mesenteric resection for cancer of the involved segment. If multiple lesions are present they may be managed by single or multiple colotomies with or without combined endoscopic cautery-snare excision, or by subtotal colectomy, dependent upon the case.

PEDUNCULATED ADENOMAS

General Principles

Adenomas become pedunculated by the traction phenomenon described earlier in this chapter. The contents of the pedicle are almost invariably limited to structures originating superficial to deep layer of the submucosa. Thus, excision at the base of the pedicle is safe and is the desired level of transection. Adenomas usually develop a pedicle only when they are 6 mm or greater in size. A rich blood supply develops in the pedicle as the polyp enlarges. These lesions can usually be totally excised with precision due to their small area of attachment to the bowel wall. It is best to excise lesions up to 8 or 9 mm in diameter by the biopsy cup technique, as this provides the best pathologic specimens. Bleeding from the wall at the base is minimal and easily controlled. Most of the remainder of the lesions can be excised by the cautery-snare technique using the equipment previously described. The snare can be passed to the level of the pedicle base in most instances. The most common obstacle to the success of this procedure is a large polyp head. This difficulty can be dealt with either by the use of specially formed large snare loops or by excising the summit of the lesion and then applying the loop to the remaining portion in the routine fashion.

The Selection of Rigid or Flexible Endoscopes

The majority of lesions of the left colon to the level of the splenic flexure can be reached by rigid instruments. These instruments can be passed to the lower sigmoid in 95% of cases, to the upper sigmoid and lower descending colon in 75 to 80% of cases, and to the splenic flexure in approximately 50% of cases. It is often necessary to use intravenous sedation and bowel relaxants, or even general anesthesia, to achieve the highest penetrations. We have experienced no associated bowel perforations with the use of these adjunctive measures. On the other hand, the flexible colonoscope can be passed to the level of the cecum in approximately 90% of cases, using intravenous sedation and bowel relaxants.

There is no universally applicable formula in deciding whether to remove a specific lesion distal to the splenic flexure via the rigid or the flexible endoscope. This will be influened by the specific case, by the skills and experience of the operators, and by the organizational aspects of the institution in which the patient is being treated.

It is our current practice at MSKCC to initially attempt the excision of lesions of the left colon distal to the splenic flexure through rigid instruments according to the following criteria: (1) all cases occurring in the area up to and including the lower descending colon, except when an earlier examination has indicated an unusual degree of difficulty in instrumentation; (2) those cases from the mid-descending colon to the splenic flexure where prior examination has indicated a high likelihood of success. Thus we do select excision through the flexible colonoscope for most lesions of the upper descending colon and splenic flexure area of the colon, as well as for all lesions proximal to the splenic flexure.

Excision Through Rigid Endoscopes

This is the most suitable method when applicable, as the instrumentation is relatively simple and permits a wide range of direct applications. The smaller lesions can be totally excised by appropriately sized biopsy cups, as can incidentally detected small sessile lesions. Fine snare loops can be precisely placed at the level of the pedicle base in most instances. If bleeding should occur it can be controlled by pressure or by the use of the alligator forceps as a hemostat with coagulation. The field can be easily lavaged and suctioned. All specimens can be retrieved.

Occasionally it is not possible to visualize the pedicle well at the time of snare application, either because of the position of the adenoma or because it tends to enter the instrument. Since the system is an open one the bowel cannot be inflated to improve visualization. The problem can almost always be solved successfully by carefully determining the location and size of the pedicle before placing the snare, which can then be placed and the loop approximated to the pedicle by feel. Before the current is applied, it is determined by measurement on the snare handle that the loop is of appropriate size. If a residual pedicle is present after initial excision, this is then removed.

Excision Through Flexible Endoscopes

There is extensive current literature dealing with this subject so it will not be covered here. Furthermore, continuing refinements in equipment make this such a rapidly developing field that it is best covered in current reports.

Equipment for this type of excision is costly and relatively complicated and should not be used where the simpler and more precise rigid instruments can be applied. Furthermore, problems arise with the use of flexible instruments that are not experienced with the rigid instruments, for example, with the former, it is often more difficult to lay the snare loop precisely, and equally fine wires usually cannot be used. There is no precise method available for the excision of smaller lesions. The retrieval of excised specimens can be extremely difficult and at times cannot be achieved. There is no means of controlling bleeding, should this occur, although this event is rare with good technique.

PEDUNCULATED ADENOMAS WITH CANCER

Adenocarcinoma is rare in adenomas less than 8 mm in size but increases in frequency in the larger adenomas. It is essential to detect its presence and to determine its extent accurately. It is for this reason that the pathologist must be provided with optimum material for review. The adequate management of these cases requires particularly close cooperation between the clinician and the pathologist.

In 1962, Dr. Frederick Shipkey, then in the Department of Pathology at Memorial Hospital, and I completed a review of 130 consecutive cases of pedunculated adenomas containing cancer, which were available for a follow-up of five or more years. The areas of cancer within these lesions were evaluated according to the degree of anaplasia and the extent and characteristics of invasion. The extent of invasion is shown in Table 1. Two cases showed lymphatic or vascular spread in the pedicle, and both were found to have regional node metastases. These were also the only cases considered to be poorly differentiated. One of the cases with spread to the base of the pedicle was also found to have regional node metastases. It has since been our practice to treat as fully malignant tumors those cases in which any of the following three criteria are met: (1) The cancer is poorly differentiated; (2) there is lymphatic or vascular spread in the pedicle distinctly separate from the primary site of the cancer; and (3) the invasive cancer extends to the level of transection at the base of the pedicle. These cases represent only approximately

Table 1. Adenoma Carcinoma—Extent of Invasion; 130 Pedunculated Lesions[a]

In situ	53	40.8%
Indeterminate superficial	19	14.5%
Summit pedicle	47	36.2%
Midpedicle	6	4.6%
Base pedicle	5	3.9%
	130 =	100.0%
Lymphatic or vascular spread in pedicle	2 . =	1.5%

[a] F. Shipkey, R. Hertz, unpublished data.

5% of those containing cancer. We would be most reluctant to advise abdominoperineal resection in the case of a low-lying lesion which demonstrated extension to the base of the pedicle.

COLOTOMY AND COLOSCOPY

Colotomy and coloscopy is a diagnostic technique for use in the examination of the entire colonic mucosa at the time of planned transabdominal excision of a colonic adenoma. The method to be used for the removal of visualized lesions is selected according to the principles previously stated. Flexible colonoscopy has largely obviated the need for this procedure, although it should remain a valuable part of the surgeon's armamentarium. Its current application is essentially limited to those cases that cannot be managed with flexible instruments, either because passage cannot be accomplished through the entire colon, or because of the presence of a distal extensive tumor.

The method consists of two or three colotomies performed in the line of a tinea, with excision of previously demonstrated lesions, and the passage of a sigmoidoscope through the colon, with further excisions as indicated. The technique will result in low morbidity if careful attention is directed towards preoperative preparation of the colon and intraoperative screening and cleansing of the field. It is practical to alter this technique by transanal passage of a flexible colonoscope after mobilization of the area that could not previously be maneuvered. It is also advisable to mobilize those angulated fixed areas that had precluded colonoscopy, so that it may be possible to accomplish colonoscopy on follow-up at a later date.

The results of colotomy and coloscopy performed at Memorial Hospital have been reviewed periodically, and the results of these procedures were essentially constant (6–8). More mucosal lesions than those demonstrated on barium enema were found in approximately 50% of cases. Cancer, varying from in situ to fully invasive types, was found in approximately 25% of those cases that had been thought to be benign adenomas. In many instances the cancer occurred in an incidentally detected, previously undiagnosed lesion. The procedure was found to carry an acceptable, low complication rate. An unpublished review of 247 cases without associated major colon resection showed a mortality rate of 0.4% and an incidence of symptomatic peritonitis of 2%. These results include patients with both pedunculated and sessile lesions (Fig. 5).

MULTIPLE POLYPOSIS

Multiple Polyps of the Colon

There are patients with multiple adenomas of the rectum and colon whose cases do not fall into the classical variants of familial multiple polyposis; they lack the traits of autosomal dominance and degree of hereditary penetration characteristic of the latter. These cases of multiple adenomas occur more often than the classical cases and are difficult to define since they demonstrate all possible variants in age of first clinical presentation, number and location of lesions, and extent of familial history.

These cases vary so greatly the one from the other that no overall plan of management can be outlined. The basic plan of continuing care should be that of excision of all

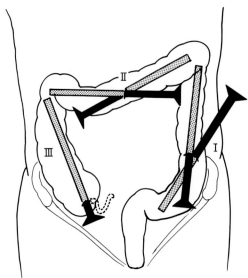

Figure 5. Colotomy and coloscopy: a sigmoidoscope is shown being passed through two invasions in the axis of the tinea and through the enlarged appendiceal stump, for visualization of the entire colon. If prior appendectomy has been performed, minimal mobilization of the hepatic flexure permits examination to the cecum through position II.

lesions using the sigmoidoscope and colonoscope, and a follow-up routine similar to that discussed in Chapters 2 and 14 for patients with adenomas. If there is difficulty in control by these methods, subtotal colectomy with ileosigmoidostomy at a level of approximately 20 cm from the anal verge is usually the treatment of choice. This allows a sufficient length of distal colon and rectum for good function, and yet control of adenomas in the residual segment is usually easily achieved by periodic sigmoidoscopy and excision. A longer segment of functional large gut is retained in these cases than is recommended for cases of familial polyposis, since the intensity of adenoma formation is usually much less than in the latter.

Familial Multiple Polyposis of the Colon

The term familial multiple polyposis of the colon includes only those cases where there is a family history consistent with the penetrance of autosomal dominance. Patients with this condition have long been known to be at extremely high risk for the development of cancer of the large gut at a relatively young age. Most of these cases show diffuse polyposis of the colon and rectum, but a small group have sparing or minimal involvement of the rectal segment. Several variants of polyposis, with associated characteristics, have been described. These secondary features do not usually influence the central problems of the management of polyposis of the large gut and the prevention and early detection of cancer of this site. A periodic search should also be made for polyps of the upper gastrointestinal tract and periampullary cancers, which occur more frequently in this disease complex. These cases have been managed by most surgeons using the sphincter-preserving operations of ileoproctostomy or ileosigmoidostomy, followed by periodic examination of the remaining segment, with cautery excision of adenomas as they develop, and subsequent excision of the segment with ileostomy, if control of the polyposis cannot be achieved or if cancer develops therein. It has been thought that these procedures provide a safe method for prolonged or indefinite postponement of sacrifice of anal sphincteric function.

The reports of Moertel, Hill, and Adson (9,10), however, cast serious doubt upon the wisdom of preserving the rectal segment in those cases showing diffuse polyposis of the colon and rectum, because in 59% of their cases, subsequent cancer of this segment developed. On the other hand, Bussey (11), reporting on the St. Marks Hospital experience with 89 cases with ileorectal anastomosis, found only two patients who developed carinomas, and these were detected at an early and presumably curative stage. The experience with sphincter-preserving procedures in this disease at the Memorial Sloan-Kettering Cancer Center has recently been reviewed by Harvey, Quan, and Stearns (12). Twenty-nine cases were suitable for evaluation of the method. Four patients developed cancer in the segment. Two cases were detected at an early stage on follow-up and resection for control of the disease was performed. Two patients developed fatal cancer: in one patient, the cancer developed in the blind pouch of an end-to-side ileoproctostomy; the other cancer was in a patient who had failed to report for follow-up examinations for over eight years. In three other patients, excision of the rectal stump was necessary because of uncontrollable polyposis. The authors concluded that the sphincter-preserving procedure is safe and advisable but that total coloproc-tectomy should be performed in patients for whom the quality of follow-up is questiona-ble and for whom control of rectal polyposis is unsatisfactory, particularly in those patients forty years of age or older.

It is our practice at MSKCC to perform the anastomosis of the ileoproctostomy in patients with familial multiple polyposis at approximately 10–12 cm from the anal verge. Before colonic resection is carried out, the rectal segment is cleared of polyps at the level of the planned anastomosis. Follow-up with excision of polyps as indicated is then staged at six-month intervals. If these patients require subsequent resection of the rectal segment with ileostomy, they are potential candidates for the Koch continent ileostomy in the pure forms of polyposis. However, the use of this procedure is contrain-dicated in Gardner's syndrome, because of the likelihood of subsequent desmoid forma-tion with small-bowel compromise.

REFERENCES

1. Gilbertsen VA: Proctosigmoidoscopy and polypectomy in reducing the incidence of rectal cancer. *Cancer* 34:936, 1974.

2. Grinnell RS, Lane N: Benign and malignant adenomatous polyps and papillary adenomas of the colon and rectum. An analysis of 1856 tumors in 1335 patients. *Surgery* 106:519, 1958.

3. Helwig EB: Adenomas and the pathogenesis of cancer of the colon and rectum. *Dis Colon Rectum* 2:5, 1959.

4. Muto T, Bussey HJR, Morson BC: The evolution of cancer of the colon and rectum. *Cancer* 36:2251, 1975.

5. Quan SH, Castro EB: Papillary adenomas (villous tumors) a review of 215 cases. *Dis Colon Rectum* 14:267, 1971.

6. Deddish MR, Hertz RE: Colotomy and coloscopy in management of mucosal polyps and cancer of the colon. *Am J Surg* 90:846, 1955.

7. Deddish MR, Hertz RE: Coloscopy in the treatment of mucosal polyps of the colon. *Surg Clin N Am* Oct. 1957, p. 1287.

8. Deddish MR, Hertz RE: Colotomy and Coloscopy in the management of neoplasms of the colon. *Dis Colon Rectum* 2:133, 1959.

9. Moertel CG, Hill JR, Adson MA: Surgical management of multiple polyposis: The problem of cancer in the retained segment. *Arch Surg* 100:521, 1970.

10. Moertel CG, Hill JR, Adson MA: Management of multiple polyposis of the large bowel. *Cancer* 28:160, 1971.

11. Bussey HJR: *Familial Polyposis Coli.* Baltimore, Johns Hopkins Univ Press, 1975.

12. Harvey JC, Quan SH, Stearns MW: Management of familial polyposis with preservation of the rectum. *Surgery* 84:476, 1978.

6
Adenocarcinoma

Maus W. Stearns, Jr.

Treatment of adenocarcinoma of the colon and rectum with the intent to cure is a surgical procedure. In the majority of patients this requires a well-executed surgical resection designed as a cancer operation, not one developed primarily to remove inflammatory disease of the bowel.

PREOPERATIVE EVALUATION

Preoperative medical evaluation of the patient as a surgical risk has been discussed in chapter 3. However, a number of factors regarding the patient are important in the determination of the proper treatment, whether for cure or palliation. Physical examination demonstrating supraclavicular, hepatic, multiple abdominal, or cul-de-sac masses usually indicates an incurable situation, as does roentgenographic demonstration of multiple pulmonary metastases. Laboratory tests, indicating elevated alkaline phosphatase or transaminase in particular, may suggest liver metastases. Carcinoembryonic antigen elevations do not necessarily indicate metastatic disease.

The examination of the tumors themselves, particularly of those that are palpable within the rectum, is critical to determine size, location, and degree of fixation or extension into adjacent rectovaginal septum, prostate, seminal vesicles, or pelvic wall. A clinically fixed or partially fixed tumor usually indicates the need for preoperative radiation therapy.

Preoperative intravenous pyelography is essential for the demonstration of bilateral kidney function, which may be a critical issue during the course of the subsequent operation. Occasionally preoperative cystoscopy is indicated, particularly for the anteriorly situated tumor where there may be questionable invasion of the bladder.

PREOPERATIVE BOWEL PREPARATION

The most important consideration in bowel preparation is the provision of a mechanically clean bowel. This can be accomplished in the patient by saline catharsis for three or four days and a clear liquid diet for two days before the operation. In the uncomplicated normal-risk patient, 30 cc of concentrated solution of magnesium sulfate three times a day is an effective saline catharsis. Castor oil (60 cc) is given the afternoon before surgery. This preparation is modified when there are symptoms of partial obstruction or when the patient is feeble or debilitated; in such cases, relatively small amounts of mineral oil and milk of magnesia are substituted. Occasionally, preoperative parenteral nutrition is necessary for optimum preparation. In recent years, antibiotics have been added to the saline catharsis preparation during the last 48 hours of treatment. Currently we use Kanamycin. Antibiotics are not added when an abdominoperineal resection with a permanent colostomy is anticipated. At MSKCC, we do not believe that antibiotics are as essential as a mechanically clean bowel.

We see very few patients initially at our institution who are so completely obstructed that they require a preliminary colostomy. Most patients who are partially obstructed can be managed by small doses of mineral oil and milk of magnesia along with a liquid diet, allowing preparation for a definitive procedure. In the infrequent case where a colostomy is necessary, considerable thought should be given to the location in the colon, since a three-stage procedure can often be avoided by locating the colostomy near enough to the obstructing tumor so that it can be removed at the same time the primary tumor is resected.

PRINCIPLES OF CANCER SURGERY OF THE BOWEL

The basic principles of cancer surgery of the colon and rectum are the same as for cancer in any site. There should be a wide local resection of the tumor-bearing segment of bowel along with as wide removal of the lymphatic drainage of that particular segment as is feasible. These resections should be performed with a minimum of cancer-cell contamination. In practice wide removal of the colonic mesentery containing the lymphatic drainage of the various segments of the bowel also effects a wide removal of the segment of the bowel bearing the tumor.

The measures used to minimize cancer-cell contamination are in essence those employed to avoid bacterial contamination. Among these measures are full-thickness protection over the entire abdominal wall incision by a double lap pad with a sheet of rubber between. This is placed before the tumor is palpated and not removed until after the tumor has been resected. Thorough abdominal exploration should be carried out before the tumor is approached or palpated. The tumor is isolated by packing the remaining viscera away with laparotomy pads. The tumor itself is manipulated as little as possible. We do palpate the tumor to determine operability and any other problems that might be involved in resection. Contaminated gloves are washed frequently. After resection of the tumor the tumor bed is irrigated. Contaminated packs are changed. Gloves are washed. Before performing an anastomosis, crushed tissue is excised and the contents of the proximal and distal bowel segments are aspirated. The mucosa and ends of the open bowel are swabbed with whatever skin preparation we use. We remove and replace all contaminated drapes and gloves before closing the abdominal wall.

THE COLON

An arbitrary but useful definition of the colon is the intraperitoneal portion of the large bowel proximal to 11 cm from the anal verge. The consideration of this portion of the large bowel separately from the rectum is justified, as the management of tumors here presents quite different problems from those of the rectum. Similarly, the chance for survival following resections for lesions here is considerably better than in patients with cancers of the rectum.

The lymphatic drainage of the colon has been well described by Rouviere (5) (Fig. 1). In summary, the lymphatics of the colon drain centrally in the mesentery, following the vascular supply. On the right side of the colon the vascular supply arises from the superior mesenteric system. On the left side the lymphatics follow the inferior mesenteric vascular channels. Thus lesions of the right colon require resections that include the entire mesentery down to the vascular origin from the superior mesenteric artery and vein. In some patients, beside the ileocolic, right colic, and midcolic vessels, an additional branch of the superior mesenteric separate from the middle colic supplies the distal transverse colon and splenic flexure. Similarly, on the left side of the colon the mesentery should be mobilized so that it can be transected at the level of the inferior mesenteric artery origin from the aorta and at the inferior mesenteric vein as it goes up under the duodenum. These resections should be performed by meticulous dissection which may occasionally be helped by transillumination of the mesentery (Fig. 2).

The operations are designed to remove these lymphatic areas. Thus, right hemicolectomy includes the entire right colon and its mesentery to the origin of the vessels from the superior mesentery (Fig. 3). For cecal lesions an additional 10–20 cm of the terminal ileum should be included to ensure an adequate removal of the lymphatics along the ileocecal vessels. For lesions in the cecum the dissection need not include the entire midcolic vasculature, but should include the right branches of the midcolic. For

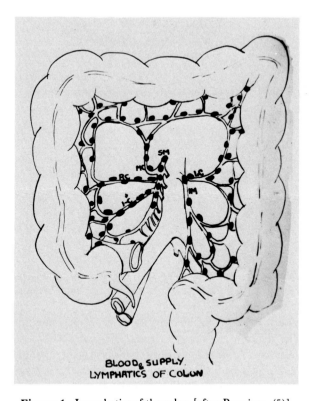

Figure 1. Lymphatics of the colon [after Rouviere, (5)].

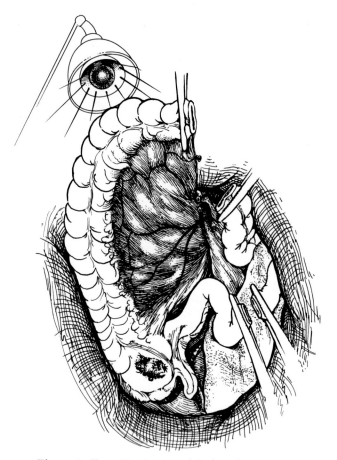

Figure 2. Transillumination of the bowel mesentery.

lesions of the hepatic flexure not as much of the terminal ileum need be removed, but the entire midcolic vascular drainage should be reached. For lesions of the midtransverse colon the procedure should be an extended right hemicolectomy, including the splenic flexure and part of the descending colon.

Right hemicolectomy has been a standard procedure for many years. Rosi (4) suggested left hemicolectomy for left-colon lesions (Fig. 4). An exception to left hemicolectomy for left-colon lesions is a lesion in the distal sigmoid (Fig. 5). Here removal of the mesentery up to the origin of the inferior mesenteric artery and the vein as it goes under the duodenum effectively accomplishes removal of the lymphatic drainage. The remaining left colon need not be removed, since the lymphatic drainage is central along the inferior mesenteric vessels, not along the marginal vessels. Paramedian incisions are preferred.

Right hemicolectomy is begun by incising the parietal peritoneum well away away from the tumor. The incision is extended proximally and distally as far as is needed. Exposure can be increased by traction on the bowel without manipulating the tumor itself (Fig. 6). The site of bowel transection is selected early and appropriate clamps applied. Further dissection mobilizes the bowel and mesentery, allowing identification of the branches from the superior mesenteric vessels, which are clamped, ligated, and cut. The bowel itself can be divided whenever it is convenient, to make the dissection easier to perform. The cut ends are covered with a small pad after being swabbed with skin antiseptic. When the resection has been completed and the specimen removed, the bed is irrigated with sterile distilled water, gloves are washed, and contaminated packs are replaced.

On the left side, inferior mesenteric vessels may be isolated more readily and directly without preliminary mobilization of the bowel. However, it is technically easier for most surgeons to mobilize the bowel and identify the origin of the vascular pedicle. Anastomoses are open, end-to-end, with a continuous over-and-over inner layer of atraumatic chromic catgut and an outer layer of interrupted silk. The outer layer of interrupted silk is placed without tying. The crushed ends of bowel are removed by incising the normal bowel tissue along the clamp. The lumen is aspirated and swabbed (Fig. 7) and the outer layer is then tied. The inner layer of chromic catgut suture is started in the center of the posterior wall and carried as an over-and-over suture to the lateral corner, where it is locked. Another similar suture is run to the opposite corner. The inner layer is completed by a Connel type of suture on the anterior wall. The two sutures are tied in the middle. An outer layer of interrupted silk completes the anastomosis.

On the right side, when there is a large defect in the mesentery, it may be closed. On the left side, the defect in the mesentery is seldom open and usually need not be repaired. Appendices epiploicae tacked over the actual suture line provide peritoneal protection.

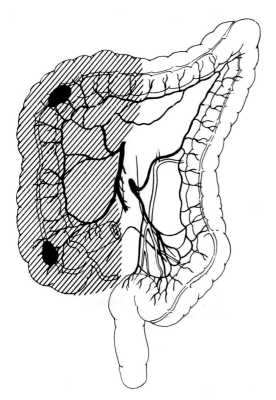

Figure 3. Extent of right hemicolectomy.

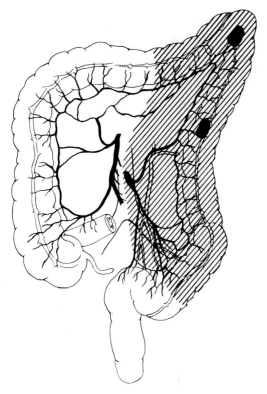

Figure 4. Extent of left hemicolectomy.

Results

One of the most significant studies regarding long-term survival following resections for cancer of the colon was reported by Turnbull et al in 1967 (10). They compared their results using the "no-touch isolation" technique with the results following "conventional surgery" performed by other surgeons at the Cleveland Clinic. One of the unique values of this report is that it compares end results in the same institution with the same patient population following operations performed by different methods. The survival rate for Dukes' A, B, and C lesions following "no-touch" resections was 68%, while for those following conventional surgery the rate was 52%. More significantly, patients with Dukes' C lesions treated by Turnbull had a five-year survival rate of 57.8%, while for those treated by conventional methods the rate was 28%.

In a review of our patients at MSKCC, using similar statistical methods of reporting (9), we found that our five-year survival rate was almost identical to that of Turnbull (Table 1). We did have a slightly lower five-year survival rate in those with Dukes' C lesions. Our series included a number of patients excluded from Dr. Turnbull's series. Almost half of the resections in our series were performed by residents under direct supervision of an attending surgeon. One-quarter of the patients in our series were typical city hospital patients from the James Ewing Hospital. In view of the similarity of our results and the fact that we had not used the "no-touch" technique, we reviewed Turnbull's original article to identify similarities in procedures. In this article there are diagrams of the operations performed. The "conventional operation" indicates a limited

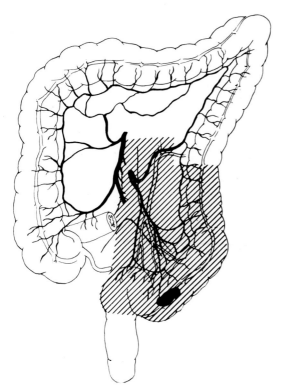

Figure 5. Sigmoid resection.

segmental resection with little mesentery included, an operation one might do for an isolated diverticulitis (Fig. 8). The diagram of the "no-touch" operation indicates a left hemicolectomy with a wide resection of the mesentery to the origin of the inferior mesenteric vessels (Fig. 9). Hence, it is our conviction that the most important consideration of Turnbull's operation is the adequacy of his cancer resection. What Turnbull performs with the "no-touch" technique we accomplish with a thorough resection of the lymphatics of the mesentery.

Table 1. Comparative Survival Rates
for Colon Cancer[a]

	Turnbull 1950–1964		Memorial Hospital 1949–1959	
	No.	*5-year[a] survival (%)*	*No.*	*5-year[b] survival (%)*
A, B and C	460	68.85	518	69.25
C	153	57.84	185	52.19

[a] Reproduced with permission from *Cancer* 28:165–169, 1971.

[b] Life table without correction for normal mortality expectation.

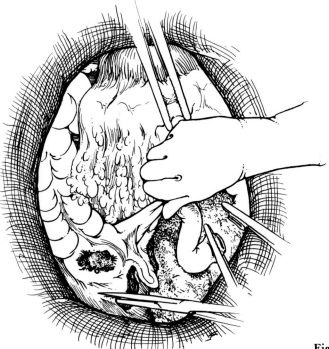

Figure 6. Traction mobilization.

THE RECTUM

The problems of surgical treatment of cancer of the rectum are quite different than those of the intraperitoneal colon because of the bony pelvis, which limits the extent of resection possible (Fig. 10). Thus, the principle of wide local removal of the cancer-bearing bowel segment is subject to severe limitations by the anatomy of the pelvic rectum. In the upper rectum it is possible to obtain a substantial margin of bowel below the tumor. This is not possible in the lower rectum, where the bowel passes through the levator and anal sphincter muscles, unless these structures are removed.

Furthermore, there are important differences in the lymphatic drainage of the rectum. In the upper half, that is, above 6 cm from the anal verge, the lymphatic drainage is cephalad along the superior hemorrhoid into the inferior mesenteric system. In the lower rectum, below 6–7 cm, the lymphatic drainage may be cephalad, caudad, or lateral. This difference in lymphatic drainage is another basis for the variation in surgical approach to lesions of the upper or lower rectum.

For lesions of the upper rectum (above 6 cm) sphincter-preserving procedures are justified if they can be done technically. They can be carried out with an adequate margin below the tumor and as much of the potential lymphatic drainage will be removed as in a resection where the distal bowel, levators, and the perineal tissue are removed. For tumors of the lower rectum, to obtain an adequate margin and remove potential lymphatic drainage distally as well as cephalad, the classical Miles' abdominoperineal resection is indicated.

As a result of these considerations, at MSKCC we have used three basic operations for cancer of the rectum. Anterior resection with primary anastomosis and "pull-

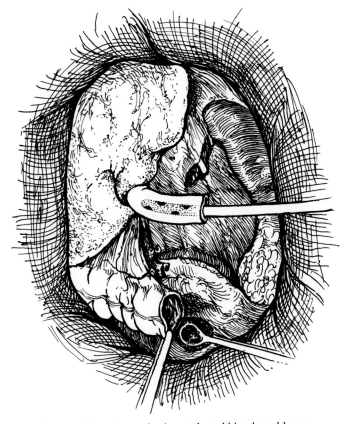

Figure 7. Suction aspiration and swabbing bowel lumen.

through" of the Bacon-Babcock type of abdominoperineal proctosigmoidectomy are sphincter-preserving procedures used for lesions in the upper rectum. The Miles' type abdominoperineal resection has been standard for the distal rectum and for some lesions of the upper rectum for which a sphincter-preserving procedure cannot be carried out for various anatomic or technical reasons (6).

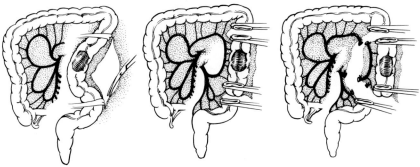

Figure 8. Conventional technic (reproduced with permission from Ann. Surg. 166:420, 1967).

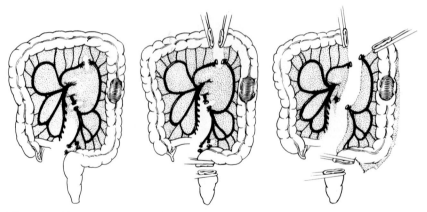

Figure 9. No-touch Isolation technic (reproduced with permission from Ann. Surg. 166:420, 1967).

It is basic that the same abdominal and pelvic dissection is indicated for any type of resection for cancer of the rectum regardless of the cancer's location. After entering and exploring the abdomen and placing the patient in deep Trendelenburg position, the intestines are packed in the upper abdomen. The dissection is begun by identifying the ureters and incising the peritoneum over the ureters into the pelvis and cephalad to the duodenoum. By blunt and sharp dissections the tissues of the mesosigmoid are then freed from the common iliac arteries up to the bifurcation, thus allowing elevation and iden-

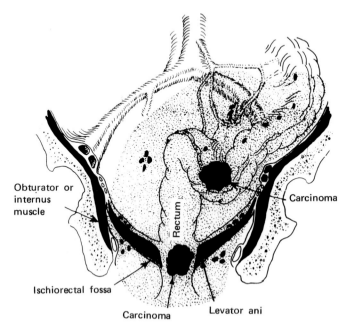

Obturator or
internus
muscle

Carcinoma

Rectum

Ischiorectal fossa

Levator ani

Carcinoma

Figure 10. Anatomical relations, pelvis. Stippled area indicates extent of resection. Heavy dots indicate lymph glands.

tification of the pedicle containing the inferior mesenteric artery and vein and mesenteric lymphatics. The peritoneal incision is then continued across the midline uniting the two sides at the level of the lower border of the duodenum near the origin of the inferior mesenteric artery. The tissues around the vessels are stripped caudad along the pedicle until the inferior mesenteric artery and vein are identified at or close to the origin from the aorta. An additional stripping of the tissue from the aorta and vena cava up to the lower border of the pancreas may be added. The vessels are identified, clamped, doubly tied, and transected.

In the ordinary good-risk patient the dissection is then continued by dissecting the tissue from the aortic bifurcation, exposing the common iliac vein down to the presacral fascia. By blunt and sharp dissection the tissues along the common iliac, external iliac, and internal iliac are freed, allowing further mobilization into the presacral space. Once the presacral space has been freed the hand is passed into the pelvis, keeping the back of the fingers against the presacral fascia. By a sweeping, cradle-type motion the remaining mesentery of the rectum is freed from the underlying fascia. The dissection is facilitated by keeping the lateral extent of dissection comparable to the lowermost portion. If one continues only posteriorly one may encounter bleeding, the source of which cannot be visualized. Anteriorly the peritoneal incisions are connected across the midline either on the back of the vagina or on the seminal vesicles and prostate, which are then freed by blunt and sharp dissection from the rectum. In the depth of the pelvis it is advantageous to identify Waldeyer's fascia, which comes from the back of the rectum onto the lower sacrum by tenting it with long forceps and then incising it. The dissecting hand can then be inserted, allowing considerably more mobilization of the rectum in the hollow of the pelvis. The lateral stalks containing the middle hemorrhoids may be transected without prior clamping. If bleeding persists, the vessels may be individually clamped and tied.

After mobilization of the rectum has been completed, the type of procedure to be employed is finally decided. As a practical guide, if two fingers can be placed below the palpable border of the tumor and a right-angle clamp placed below them, and if a transection distal to the clamp can then be performed, with enough rectal segment left to do an anastomosis, an anterior resection should be done. If there is an adequate margin below the tumor but a clamp cannot be placed with an adequate stump, one should consider a pull-through. If there is no adequate stump an abdominoperineal resection should be done. The abdominal wall is closed is 30 or 28 steel wire applied in a Tom-Jones–type suture that effects peritoneal and fascial approximation. The skin is closed with metal clips.

Anterior Resection

When an anterior resection is to be done sutures are placed in the lateral tissue of the distal stump after placing the distal clamp, before dividing the distal bowel. These sutures give support to the rectal stump and control bleeding from the inferior hemorrhoidal. A right-angle Wertheim hysterectomy clamp or a Pott's clamp have proved most practical for this purpose in the low rectum. As much of the bowel should be included as is feasible, but complete occlusion with the clamp is not always possible. A single-thickness laparotomy pad in the pelvis protects the ureters and iliac vessels. The bowel is divided below the clamp with a right-angle knife or scissors and the specimen is removed. Before this step the sigmoid and its mesentery will have been divided. Allen clamps are satisfactory for this purpose in the proximal bowel. The proximal bowel may be freed of fat in preparation for anastomosis before the bowel is divided.

After removal of the specimen, bleeding in the distal stump is controlled, the rectal stump is aspirated, and the lumen and ends swabbed with skin preparation. The pelvis should be irrigated with distilled water. Laparotomy pads are packed tightly in the pelvis to control oozing and are left there while the proximal bowel is prepared for anastomosis. Incision of the lateral parietal peritoneum usually gives enough mobilization of the proximal sigmoid and descending colon to allow approximation of the proximal colon to the rectal stump for the anastomosis. If this step is insufficient, mobilization of the splenic flexure is necessary.

The anastomosis is performed by placing a row of interrupted atraumatic chromic sutures posteriorly. One method is to place an angle suture on each side and then simply suture to divide the posterior walls repeatedly until enough sutures are in place. After they have all been placed, the bowel ends are approximated and the knots are tied in the lumen of the bowel. The anterior layer is completed with either interrupted chromic catgut sutures or a continuous running suture to approximate the bowel edges, and then a second row of interrupted chromic catgut is placed. Reinforcing sutures are used where possible.

There are differences in procedures of draining the pelvis following low-anterior resection, varying from simple cigarette drains removed after 24 hours to drains that remain in place for ten to twelve days. Hemovac or Shirley sump suction is used frequently. The reason for this variety of methods is that none is completely satisfactory. Early experience with the intestinal stapler suggests that this implement may be very useful if adequate distal rectal segment remains after completion of the resection.

A substantial number of low anastomoses are protected with proximal transverse colostomies. This procedure is frequently indicated because of the poor general condition of the patient, particularly those of advanced years, since the elderly do not tolerate infection well. A colostomy is strongly indicated for a woman whose uterus has been removed, where the vaginal stump closure is at the same level as the anastomosis. Other indications are a poorly prepared bowel or a less than technically satisfactory anastomosis.

Pull-Through

In considering the choice of procedure, a pull-through may be indicated early in the course of mobilization. With this in mind, umbilical tape is used instead of a clamp on the proximal bowel at the point of eventual transsection. The rest of the pelvic dissection is the same as for any resection of the rectum. When it is finally decided that a pull-through is to be performed, it is essential to mobilize the descending colon more thoroughly than one might for an anterior resection. Often this means mobilizing the splenic flexure. The abdomen is closed unless there is a question of available length. The patient placed in a lithotomy position. A posterior sphincterotomy to the tip of the coccyx has reduced the sloughing of the protruding bowel segment. A purse-string suture is placed through the lower rectal mucosa. The mucocutaneous junction is completely incised and the mucosa of the anal canal is freed from the underlying musculature until the pelvis is entered.

Mobilization from the puborectalis allows the bowel to be drawn through the canal until the umbilical tape appears. The distal bowel is transected and removed. The proximal colon is then fixed by placing a rubber catheter into its lumen, which is then tied with an umbilical tape. Appendices epiploica are sutured to the skin. The protruding bowel is covered with vaseline gauze. The rubber tube is removed in three to four days. The pelvis is drained by a generous stab wound through the perineum through which ischiorectal fossa and a large rubber drain are inserted into the pelvis.

Abdominoperineal Resection

This section is based on a previous report by the author (7). The sigmoid is divided at the same level between Payr clamps. After completing pelvic dissection, the redundant sigmoid and upper rectum are removed by transecting the rectum as low as is convenient, using either umbilical tapes or Wolfson DeMartel at point of division. The peritoneal floor is usually reconstructed after mobilizing the peritoneum from the pelvic wall and bladder by a running chromic suture interrupted several times. If the pelvic peritoneum cannot be closed, a rubber dam packed with gauze is introduced in the perineal phase to keep the small bowel out of the pelvis. The colostomy is formed by bringing the sigmoid through the abdominal incision about two-thirds of the way between the symphysis and umbilicus, leaving the Payr clamp to support the colostomy.

The patient is then placed in extreme lithotomy position. The perineal phase is started by placing a purse string to close the anal canal. A shield-shaped incision is made from the ischial tuberosities bilaterally to the tip of the coccyx posteriorly and to an arbitrary point on the perineum, depending on whether the patient is a man or woman. In women, the rectovaginal septum is separated. In men the incision is made at the level of the transverse perineus muscle. Incisions are deepened along the ischiotuberosity until the levator muscles are identified. Posteriorly the incision exposes the tip of the coccyx. After the levators are identified, an incision is made in front of the coccyx entering the pelvis. The levator muscles are then retracted medially between the fingers of the left hand and, with the scissors, the attachment of the levators is cut from the pelvic wall. When this has been completed on both sides, the rectal stump is brought out through the posterior wound. By sharp dissection along the pelvic side of the rectum it is removed from the vagina or the prostate. Care must be taken to avoid the membranous urethra in the male.

After the specimen has been removed bleeding is controlled. Terramycin powder is placed in the pelvis and a gauze-filled rubber glove is placed in the pelvic defect and held in place with silk sutures through the perineal skin. These sutures are removed in two to three days, and the packing is gradually removed from the rubber glove over the next three or four days.

Results

In Table 2 our five-year survival rates are shown for patients having curative resection for cancer of the upper and lower rectum with and without nodal metastases. It is evident that the results are poorer in cases involving the distal rectum, regardless of the presence or absence of nodal metastases. Table 3 shows our use of these three procedures in cancer of the upper and lower rectum. These results show that in cases of

Table 2. Survival and Location of Primary Regional Nodes, 1957–1967

	Negative		Positive	
	Below 6 cm	–11 cm	Below 6–11 cm	6–11 cm
Number resections	112	193	61	129
Indeterminate	20	30	12	12
5-year survivors	67	130	17	51
Cancer after 5 years	8	12	4	8
5-year survival %				
Overall[b]	60	67	28	40
Determinate[c]	73	80	35	44
N.E.C.[d]	64	72	26.5	37

[a] Reproduced with permission from *Cancer* 34:969–971, 1974.

[b] Overall: All five-year survivors (all curative resections).

[c] Determinate: All five-year survivors (all curative resections) minus those dying postoperatively, those dying in less than five years of other causes with no evidence of cancer, and those lost to followup in less than five years with no evidence of cancer.

[d] N.E.C. (no evidence of cancer): All five-year survivors minus those with cancer after five years (determinate patients).

lesions in the distal rectum, 90% of the patients were treated by abdominoperineal resection, whereas in cases involving the upper rectum, more than three-quarters of the patients had undergone some type of a sphincter-preserving procedure, usually an anterior resection.

Table 4 presents the survival rates following each of these three procedures in the

Table 3. Types of Operations Used for Rectum Cancer 1957–1967

	Level of tumor	
Operation	Below 6 cm	6–10 cm
Total resections	173	322
A.P.R.[a]	155	72
A.R.[b]	8	217
P.T.[c]	10	33
Utilization	%	%
A.P.R.	90	22.4
A.R.	4.2	67.2
P.T.	5.8	9.4

[a] A.P.R.: abdominoperineal resection, procedure of Miles.

[b] A.R.: anterior resection with anastomosis with or without proximal colostomy.

[c] P.T.: abdominoperineal "pull-through," Babcock-Bacon type.

Table 4. Comparison of Survival Rates and Type of
Operation at 6–11 cm; 1957–1967[a]

	APR	AR	PT
Total resections	72	217	33
Indeterminate	9	32	1
5-year survivors	37	120	24
Cancer after 5 years	2	10	8
5-year survival %			
Overall[b]	51	55	72
Determinate[b]	59	65	75
N.E.C.[b]	55.5	59.5	50

[a] Reproduced with permission from *Cancer* 34:969–971, 1974.

[b] See Table 2 for an explanation of these categories.

upper rectum, that is, between 6 and 11 cm. It appears that the sphincter-preserving procedures are followed by as good long-term survival as that following abdominoperineal resection.

EXTENDED RESECTIONS

The omentum should be removed with any intracolonic carcinoma which extends through the serosa. Because of the great mobility of this organ, tumor masses are frequently found within it.

Any adjacent viscera adhering to the tumor, no matter how filmy the adherence, should be resected, not freed. Direct invasion is not necessary to cause implants on an adhering bowel. However, viscera should not be removed simply because the tumor is in the same general location. Because of the finding of occult ovarian metastases in a substantial number of women who have regional node metastases, the ovaries should be removed routinely in the postmenopausal patient. In the premenopausal woman, before surgery there should be discussion concerning removal of the ovaries. The ovaries should be removed if the tumor involves the serosa or if there are probable nodal metastases.

When a colonic tumor is attached to the dome of the bladder a segmental resection should be done. The bladder repair usually does not need to be protected by a suprapubic cystotomy; an indwelling Foley catheter suffices. The entire urinary bladder needs to be removed when there is direct invasion near the trigone or substantial invasion of the prostate and seminal vesicles in men. This procedure is not indicated very often, since usually there is an inoperable lateral or posterior extension when the tumor involves the base of the bladder. The procedure may be helped along by ligation of the hypogastric arteries, which reduces blood loss. The technical details of pelvic exenteration are not greatly different from those of a resection for cancer of the rectum. The main problem is the management of the ureters following this procedure. If an abdominoperineal resection is done, implanting the ureters into the sigmoid with the establishment of a proximal colostomy has given a very satisfactory result. The distal loop is isolated from the proximal bowel 7 to 10 days after surgery by dividing the colostomy and closing the distal end, thus forming a urinary conduit and a proximal colostomy, which are not connected. If large-bowel continuity is restored by an anastomosis, a loop of ileum should be used as the ileal conduit. The ureter–intestinal anastomoses are mucosa-to-mucosa with reinforcement of the ureter to the bowel wall above it.

POSTOPERATIVE CARE

Postoperative Antibiotics

Antibiotics are indicated following the anterior resection in cases where contamination occurs and with perforated or obstructed tumors. Our current choice is ampicillin. Vibramycin is used if the patient is sensitive to penicillin. Antibiotics are given immediately before surgery and are continued for three days after the operation. If the patient is still febrile at that time, the antibiotics should be changed; the choice should be guided, when possible, by culture-sensitivity studies. (Choice of antibiotics changes periodically.)

Diet

Oral intake is withheld until peristalsis is present and there is no distension. The patient is then allowed to drink clear liquids, which are increased as tolerated; the patient progresses to a full regular diet within the next three to four days. Intravenous fluids are given as indicated.

Urinary Care

Foley catheters are inserted preoperatively in all patients having resections. The catheters are connected to straight drainage and are removed on the second or third postoperative day if pelvic surgery has not been done. Following low anterior resections or abdominoperineal resections, removal of the catheter is deferred until removal of the pack or until the patient is fully ambulatory (usually six to seven days). After removal of the Foley catheter, unless the patient is voiding normally, the residue should be checked in 24 hours. If the residue is more than 250 cc, the Foley catheter should be replaced. Urecholine 10 mg t.i.d. is started. The catheter is removed again in 48 to 72 h. A regimen of progressive clamping of the catheter has been used effectively.

Other Care

Early ambulation is encouraged, as are respiratory exercises and leg exercises in bed. "Miniheparinization," started immediately before surgery, does not seem to have created any problems and may be of value in preventing significant pulmonary emboli. The management of drains is highly individualized among surgeons. There does not appear to be any perfect method. In patients who have had an abdominoperineal resection with a permanent colostomy, the clamp is removed after 48 hours unless distension dictates earlier decompression. Transverse colostomies are opened at the bedside with a cautery within 48 hours or earlier if distension is present.

In many elderly patients and in patients who have cardiopulmonary problems a gastrostomy is performed in the operating room. This is a simple stab-wound-type gastrostomy. The catheter is brought through the abdominal wall immediately above the region where it exits from the stomach when the stomach is in its normal position and is sutured to the parietal peritoneum. The catheter is connected to straight-gravity drainage and is maintained this way until the patient's bowel activity returns, and then clamped. It need not be removed until shortly before the patient is discharged as it is often useful in periods of ileus. If a gastrostomy has not been performed, or when it does not function properly, a nasogastric tube may be necessary. These tubes need daily flushing with saline solution. When such tubes are in place it is particularly important to take respiratory physical-therapy measures to prevent pulmonary complications.

Following low anastomoses, no rectal tube, suppositories, or irrigation should be used, and rectal examination should be undertaken only if necessary and only after careful consideration.

COMPLICATIONS

Fever

Fever during the first 24 to 48 hours after surgery is almost always due to pulmonary complications and should be treated accordingly. To encourage deep breathing and coughing we find it helpful to use a scultetus binder to support the abdomen and minimize incisional discomfort. Physical-therapy respiratory exercise is most useful if instructions have been given preoperatively. They are still of value if instituted properly postoperatively. Mechanical devices to assist in deep breathing are useful, but probably less effective than simple full-coughing movement and deep-breathing exercises.

Fever occuring after 48 hours is more likely to be due to some other type of infection, and the usual methods to determine the cause should be used. The most common source following low anterior resection is some breakdown of the anastomosis or wound infection.

Anastomotic Leakage

Anastomotic leakage from an intraperitoneal colonic anastomosis is rare but is quite frequent with low extraperitoneal anastomoses. Some degree of leakage or anastomotic abscess probably occurs in a large majority of these low anastomoses, either as a pelvic cellulitis, which may be minimal and essentially asymptomatic, or as an overt fecal fistula. Anastomotic fistulas usually are self-limiting, closing spontaneously. If the patient is tolerating the fistula with or without antibiotic coverage and if he or she continues to have a substantial amount of bowel movements per rectum, no surgical intervention is necessary. Sometimes closure of the fistula can be facilitated by irrigation of the pelvis through the suprapubic fistula track by means of a small catheter with saline. This method is particularly useful when the drainage becomes purulent and pockets are suspected. The irrigations should not be started too early or vigorously because of the danger of general peritoneal contamination.

If the fistula drains more and more feces with decreasing amount of stool through the rectum over several days or increasing febrile reaction, a diverting colostomy should be seriously considered. However, this should not be done too quickly, as most of these fistulas heal spontaneously.

Postoperative Obstruction: Ileus

One of the more frequent problems encountered in the postoperative management of any bowel resection is the delay in return of bowel function. Often the differential diagnosis between postoperative obstruction or ileus is difficult. Daily auscultation of the abdomen to detect the return of peristalsis is a valuable diagnostic tool. If peristalsis simply does not return, one is faced with a prolonged ileus and conservative methods should be continued. Conservative methods consist mainly of withholding oral intake and substituting intestinal intubation, which can consist of a simple gastric tube to prevent the accumulation of swallowed air in the intestinal tract. If the ileus is more severe or unresponsive to simple intubation it may be worthwhile to try to pass a long tube. This procedure is sometimes so difficult that it is not worth the added effort.

If peristalsis returns and then disappears, associated with a rise in fever, almost certainly there is some degree of peritonitis, probably due to an anastomotic leak. Treatment of this complication requires careful evaluation. A number are self-limited and are controlled by antibiotics and continued conservative methods. However, when it is apparent that there is spreading peritonitis, which the patient (particularly an older person) cannot tolerate a proximal colostomy should be performed promptly.

If peristalsis becomes hyperactive, it is reasonably sure that some degree of obstruction is present, although again treatment has to be evaluated carefully, as a number of partial obstructions are controlled by simple conservative measures as described above. Laparotomy is rarely necessary. In all of these conditions abdominal radiography is valuable, provided the scans are used in context with the clinical condition of the patient and not as a sole diagnostic method.

Urinary Complications

Urinary complications are obviously more frequent in men, but they do occur in women as well. They are much more frequent after pelvic surgery than after intraperitoneal colonic surgery. Men who have had preoperative nocturia or frequency due to prostatic hypertrophy experience a great deal of urinary difficulty. If they have not had symptoms before surgery, conservative methods should be continued for some time, including home use of a Foley catheter if the patient is unable to void by the time he is otherwise ready to go home. The catheter should be removed in about a week. The patient removes the catheter the day before coming for the checkup. This will allow a 24-h trial. If unable to void, or if there is a high residual the Foley should again be replaced. These trials should be repeated for three to four weeks. After this period, almost all patients will be able to void normally. After several unsuccessful attempts, the patient who has had considerable problems preoperatively should be referred to a urologist, as he will probably require prostatic resection.

LOCAL PROCEDURES
IN THE TREATMENT OF CANCER OF THE RECTUM

A number of methods to treat cancer of the rectum without major resection or permanent colostomy have been described. Papillon has used high-dose, low-voltage radiotherapy for early selected cases of cancer of the rectum and has obtained very satisfactory results (3). Deddish has used local excision in a small number of carefully selected patients with equally good results (1). Electrocoagulation or fulguration has been urged as a primary and preferred method of treating rectal cancer by Madden and Kandaloft (2), with which premise we disagree.

We believe, however, that there are definite indications for local procedures (8). Villous adenomas with superficially infiltrating carcinoma that does not clinically infiltrate the muscle wall may well be treated by either local excision or fulguration. Bulky, polypoid cancer that again does not infiltrate the muscle may be treated either by local excision or by fulguration. Patients who have significant distal metastases and have a locally amenable lesion also may be treated by a local procedure. Patients who cannot or will not cope with a colostomy, if they have a locally amenable lesion, may be treated by local methods. We believe that local treatments are not justified in the usual typical infiltrating cancer in a reasonably good-risk patient. They are also unsatisfactory for patients who have an annular lesion or one that invades the rectovaginal septum.

We have not had experience with the Papillon method of high-dose, low-voltage radiation therapy. This requires special instruments, and its advantage is that it can be carried out as an outpatient procedure and does not require hospital admission. Local excisions as performed by Deddish can be carried out transanally with good visualization. The sphincter can be either dilated or transected, allowing placement of stay sutures around the lesion and removal under direct vision. The effectiveness of this method is based on careful selection. Fulguration, if it is to be done, should be carried out as described by Madden and Kandaloft (2). It should be thorough, and done under general anesthesia. It is a major operative procedure. If recurrence is found, it should be reattacked vigorously and promptly. Fulguration is not an outpatient procedure and should not be performed in a doctor's office.

REFERENCES

1. Deddish MR: Local excision. *Surg Clin N Am* 54:877–880, 1974.
2. Madden JL, Kandaloft S: Clinical evaluation of electrocoagulation in the treatment of cancer of the rectum. *Am J Surg* 122:347–352, 1971.
3. Papillon J: Endocavitary irradiation in the curative treatment of early cancer. *Dis Colon Rectum* 17:172–180, 1974.
4. Rosi PA: Hemicolectomy in the treatment of carcinoma of the left colon. Quart *Bull Northwest Univ Medical School* 23:376–383, 1949.
5. Rouviere H: *Anatomy of the Human Lymphatic System. A compendium.* Tobias, MJ (trans). Ann Arbor, Mich, Edwards Brothers, Inc, 1938, pp 188–192.
6. Stearns MW Jr: The choice among anterior resection, the pull-thru, and abdomino-perineal resection of the rectum. *Cancer* 34:969–971, 1974.
7. Stearns MW Jr: *Surg Tech Illus* 2(1):37–48, 1977.
8. Stearns MW Jr: Limitations of local treatment of carcinoma of the rectum, in Varco RL and Delaney JD (eds): *Controversy in Surgery.* Philadelphia, W. B. Saunders, 1976, chap 17, pp 401–406.
9. Stearns MW Jr, Schottenfeld D: Techniques for the surgical management of colon cancer. *Cancer* 28:165–169, 1971.
10. Turnbull RB Jr, Kyle K, Watson FR, Spratt J: Cancer of colon: The influence of "no-touch isolation" technic on survival rates. *Ann Surg* 166:420–425, 1967.

7
Surgery for Metastasis from Carcinoma of the Rectum and Colon

Fadi F. Attiyeh

It is generally assumed that when carcinoma of the colon and rectum metastasizes to distant sites the prognosis is poor and further therapy is usually aimed toward palliation. However, there are instances where metastasis is confined to one distant site, usually liver or lung, before it becomes generalized, and surgical excision can possibly render the patient free of disease for an appreciable period of time, and even cure the disease.

Over the years, here at Memorial Hospital, some of these patients were treated by surgical excision of the metastasis, with a reasonable number surviving five or more years. In the case of liver metastases, there were 25 patients between 1950 and 1976 who underwent some form of liver resection for metastases (1). Most of these were solitary and peripheral lesions that were treated with a wedge excision. The mean survival following the excision was 64 months, the median was 30 months, and the determinate 5- and 10-year survival rates were 40% and 28%, respectively. When the primary colonic lesion was a Dukes' A or B, the 5- and 10-year survival rates were 62% and 57%, respectively. When the primary tumor was a Dukes' C, the 5- and 10-year survival rates were 25% and 9%, respectively. From an earlier report about our experiences in colorectal cancer, the median survival for patients with multiple hepatic metastases was 7 months, and for those with solitary metastases that were left unresected the median survival was 19 months (2). There were no 5-year survivors in this group. Although the patients with unresected solitary lesions cannot be matched with the 25 patients who underwent liver resection (not a randomized study), they are nevertheless similar as far as the size and location of the metastasis is concerned. Wilson reported a similar experience from the Mayo Clinic, showing a 42% 5-year survival with the resection of solitary liver metastases and no 5-year survival when similar solitary lesions were left unresected (3). Our approach with hepatic metastases has been to resect solitary and peripheral metastases when detected simultaneously with the

99

primary colonic resection, if this can be accomplished easily with a wedge resection or a segmentectomy. However, if the liver metastasis is large enough to require a lobectomy, or if the medical condition of the patient at the time does not permit any form of liver resection, then the latter can be done at a second stage.

In the case of lung metastasis, there were 35 patients between 1960 and 1977 who underwent a total of 43 thoracotomies for resection of metastatic lesions (4): 15 patients had wedge excisions, 19 had lobectomies, and 1 had a pneumonectomy. The determinate 5-year survival rate for this group was 22%. The disease-free interval from the colonic resection to the pulmonary resection, the type of pulmonary resection, and the number of metastatic lesions did not correlate with survival. However, when the primary colonic lesion was a Dukes' A the 5-year survival rate was 37.5%, versus 15% in patients whose primary tumor was a Dukes' C. A solitary lung lesion in particular should be approached aggressively, since the chance that it is a primary lung cancer is as good as the chance that it is a single metastatic lesion from the colon primary. It also could be a benign pulmonary lesion. It thus becomes mandatory that a thoracotomy should be done unless there are medical contraindications for surgery.

Because of these encouraging results, we believe that surgery plays a definite role in some patients with hepatic and pulmonary metastases, especially since there is no other effective means of therapy to control the disease for an extended period of time.

REFERENCES

1. Attiyeh FF, Wanebo HJ, Stearns MW Jr: Hepatice resection for metastasis from colorectal cancer. *Dis Colon Rectum* 21(3):160, 1978.

2. Wanebo HJ, Semouglou C, Attiyeh FF, Stearns MW Jr: Surgical management of patients with primary operable colorectal cancer and synchronous liver metastases. *Am J Surg* 135:81, 1978.

3. Wilson SM, Adson MA: Surgical treatment of hepatic metastases from colorectal cancers. *Arch Surg* 111:330, 1976.

4. Attiyeh FF, McCormack PM: Resected lung metastasis from colorectal cancer. *Dis Colon Rectum* (in press).

8

Advanced Colon and Rectum Cancer

Horace W. Whiteley, Jr.

INTRODUCTION

Advanced disease of the colon and rectum presents complex problems for the patient and the physician. Over one-half of all patients afflicted with large-bowel cancer will at some time be included in this advanced-disease group. In order to provide for the intelligent care and management of these patients, a concept of the disease with particular attention to the natural history of advanced colon cancer must be developed. It is not enough to establish that an individual has advanced disease and invoke a course of therapy based on whatever current wisdom dictates. The physician must have a basic idea of what the disease consists of, what might or might not be accomplished by treatment, what measures of the treatment can be monitored, and, lastly, what results might be expected. It is the purpose of this chapter to establish guidelines and basic data to provide a concept of course of disease and a means by which effectiveness of therapy can be measured.

The patient with advanced cancer is incurable; 95% of all patients in this category will die of their disease within 36 months. What can be offered to the individual is palliation; that is, a reduction of symptoms as well as the ability to carry on normal activities. It is necessary that the involved physician have the background information at the start of his management so that an intelligent program can be developed for the patient and his family before courses of complex therapy are instituted.

DEFINITIONS

The main problem in stating a conceptual program for the care of patients with advanced large-bowel cancer is confusion in terminology. It is difficult to achieve an understanding of the problems without having a precise definition of the terms used. At the Rectum and Colon Service at Memorial Hospital, the following definitions have been found useful.

Advanced Disease

Advanced disease of the colon and rectum is cancer that cannot be surgically removed. This may be *residual cancer,* or disease that could not be removed during the initial surgical procedure; it may be *recurrent cancer* disease that becomes manifest after a curative resection; or it may be *metastatic cancer* disease that has spread by implant, lymphatics, or the bloodstream, and cannot be completely surgically excised. To restate, advanced cancer of the large bowel means nonresectable disease that may be residual, recurrent, or metastatic.

Nonresectable Disease

The key to the definition of advanced cancer is that it is a nonresectable disease. It is necessary to explore further the meaning of the term and be quite precise in its use. It is obvious that controversy may arise, since what might be resectable to one surgeon may not be to another. With our patients we try to be certain that the disease in each of these patients is indeed nonresectable, since it is basic that unless the cancer is completely excised the patient will die of the disease. There are two general areas where this concept is particularly important. In patients who are operated on elsewhere and are referred to us for evaluation, it is essential to have irrefutable evidence of nonresectability by confirmed operative and pathologic reports. Thus, confirmed pelvic-wall disease, peritoneal implants, and more than a single liver or lung metastasis are nonresectable cases. On the other hand, descriptions of extension of cancer to involve the bladder or adjacent organs, initially unresected mesenteric disease, or solitary metastasis are prime examples of disease that often can be resected. If there is any reason to hope that resectability can be obtained, that patient is reexplored.

In the typical example of presumed nonresectable pelvic disease, it is our policy to recommend preoperative radiation therapy to the pelvis with anterior and posterior ports to a level of 3000 rads before reexploration. We expect a salvage rate of 20% five-year survival in this group of patients who are referred for nonresectable disease and from whom the cancer is completely excised. A separate group of patients are those who are initially operable for cure at Memorial Hospital and in whom the cancer recurs. Although the possibility of further resection must always be considered and a preoperative course of radiation is provided, any attempt to resect a pelvic recurrence is usually not productive and is to be avoided. This decision can usually be made by digital rectal and proctosigmoidoscopy examination. If pelvic-wall disease is found in patients, reoperation is avoided because of the potential for prolonged morbidity and the loss of palliation. However, every examiner has to be particularly cautious, since there are a few patients who will develop a second primary in the pelvic colon which may simulate recurrent disease. These new cancers represent new disease and are completely resectable and curable.

SURGICAL PALLIATION

In addition to laparotomy for evaluation for resectability, there are several situations where palliation can be achieved by surgical intervention. It is basic to an overall therapeutic approach that the patient be evaluated for palliative advantage from surgery before other therapy is instituted (Table 1).

Pelvic Mass

There is an 18% incidence of ovarian metastasis in lymph-node-positive pelvic colon cancers. Although there is an increased acceptance of oophorectomy at the time of initial

Table 1. Advanced Colon and Rectum Cancer:
Surgery for Palliation

Surgery Indicated

Determination of resectability
Large abdominal mass
Bowel obstruction
Right-colon lesions

Surgery Not Indicated

Bilateral ureteral obstruction
Abdominal carcinomatosis
Impending bowel obstruction
Perineal recurrence

surgery, there are a number of women who have, when first examined, advanced disease with a large pelvic mass. These masses are usually ovarian in origin and exert considerable pressure on the bladder and rectum. Palliation can be achieved by excision of these large-mass lesions. Obviously a bilateral oophorectomy should be done. This same procedure can be applied to other areas, such as large omental implants. The overall approach is to remove symptomatic local disease whenever possible, even in the presence of distant metastasis.

Right-Colon Lesions

Most right-colon lesions should be resected for palliation, even in the presence of major metastatic problems. There are obvious exceptions where technical or medical situations take precedence, but a bypass procedure such as a side-to-side ileotransverse colostomy does not usually result in palliation. The major problems of bleeding with anemia, mass with pressure, infection, and fistula are not relieved except by resection. This concept is valid but is less frequently encountered in other areas of the intraperitoneal colon.

Obstruction

The major cause of bowel obstruction in cancer patients is adhesions. Our concept is to offer all patients with bowel obstruction one opportunity for surgical relief. Exploration for obstruction often discloses adhesions from previous surgery or a localized amount of disease that precipitated the obstruction and can be removed, reconstituting bowel continuity. This procedure is almost always effective. The prime exception is known abdominal carcinomatosis, where multiple areas of obstruction are present. The surgeon should not knowingly operate on these people, since significant relief for the patient can seldom be provided.

Principles to Consider when Dealing with Obstruction in Advanced Colon Cancer

Bypass Mucous Fistula

In instances of small-bowel obstruction due to tumor in the pelvis it is often wise to delineate the area of obstruction and bypass the obstruction without entering the tumor area. A proximal-end-to-distal-side anastomosis with the remaining end leading to the obstruction brought to the skin as a mucous fistula is a most satisfactory way of dealing with this problem. In this way the self-destructive maneuver of routing out nonresectable disease is obviated. Also, the mucous fistula allows proximal egress from the obstructed area and decreases the possibility of abscess formation.

Large-bowel Obstruction Secondary to Recurrent Pelvic Cancer

When the large bowel is obstructed within the pelvis due to pelvic-wall cancer following an anterior-resection procedure, careful consideration is necessary. While a colostomy at a distal point in the bowel is usually most satisfactory where the inferior mesenteric artery has been ligated at the initial procedure, the exteriorization and division of the left colon for colostomy and mucous fistula would leave a devascularized segment of bowel to necrose and abscess. Palliation is often lost in this situation from resulting morbidity. Also, a colostomy in an area where the mesentery is involved with tumor may lead to extension of tumor to the abdominal wall with serious complexities in care and function. The simplest and safest approach to this problem is usually a left-sided transverse colostomy without vascular interruption. If this colostomy is fashioned properly, complete diversion can be achieved.

Circumstances in which Surgery Is Not Palliative and Should Be Avoided

Bilateral Ureteral Obstruction

There is little to be gained by urinary diversion to relieve uremia when other forms of therapy such as radiation and chemotherapy have been applied to the maximum. Although uremia has been relieved by surgical manipulation, there has been no change in the course of the advanced cancer. The condition of these patients should be studied carefully before a urologic consultation is requested. Injudicious intervention in situations of intractable pain results in additional burdens on patients and their families. In the uremic patient with bilateral ureteral obstruction, examination by ill-considered ureteral catherization is to be condemned, since it often results in perforation or infection. Unless there is reasonable evidence to indicate that bilateral ureteral obstruction is due to causes other than advanced pelvic cancer, ureteral manipulation is contraindicated.

Impending Obstruction

Another procedure to be condemned and avoided is the colostomy for impending obstruction. If the patient is obstructed, a colostomy is needed for relief. However, it is not always wise to anticipate an impending obstruction and perform a procedure that may be unnecessary. In cases of advanced disease colostomies do not function properly and the cancer may take other paths, which obviates the need for colostomy.

Pelvic Recurrence

A major problem in the treatment of advanced disease is the recurrence of pelvic cancer following abdominoperineal resection. Such a recurrence is to be suspected when the symptoms of pelvic pressure, sciatic-nerve-root pain, and a perineal mass occur. These symptoms are a result of disease in the pelvic wall lymphatics, which progresses in the pelvis and may finally appear as a palpable tumor in the perineum. The palpable disease represents only the "tip of the iceberg." Any attempt at surgery is unproductive and incision into the mass even for biopsy produces a fungating perineal tumor mass. Palliative methods of treatment, such as pelvic radiation, are more effective. Rarely, a true implant that appears in the perineum can be locally removed, but this is unusual and presents a different clinical picture.

CLASSIFICATION OF ADVANCED DISEASE

Once the surgical considerations of the patient with advanced colon cancer have been resolved, it becomes necessary to further evaluate the individual as to the state of involvement of the disease and the patient's response to the disease. Here an understanding of the natural history of advanced colon cancer is necessary. It is no longer satisfactory to substantiate nonresectable disease and then provide a cookbook form of therapy, even if this is in present-day vogue. Also, it is exceedingly important to understand what may be accomplished with advanced cancer in general as well as in the individual patient. To accomplish this we have developed a systematized classification so patients with like forms of the disease can be compared. There are two elements to our classification.

Patterns of Disease

Advanced colon cancer as a progressive disease has a tendency to follow certain clinical forms (1). These forms are quite separate, with different symptoms, and a characteristic cause and method of disease. The different clinical forms are referred to as patterns of disease. They are reserved entirely for the advanced state. There are four separate patterns: local pattern, hepatic pattern, intraabdominal pattern, and generalized pattern. These patterns are separate clinical entities, with individuals in one group having a different course than individuals in another pattern group. The patterns have unique survival patterns and theoretically should suggest various treatment courses.

Local Pattern

The local pattern is disease present at a certain site in the abdomen or pelvis that is not resectable (Fig. 1). Local disease causes symptoms by local progression and invasion. Metastatic disease may be present, but it does not represent the major symptoms or course of the disease. The typical example of this pattern is pelvic-wall disease, either residual or recurrent, which produces pelvic symptoms, including sciatic root pain. The disease progresses with adjacent organ involvement, in some cases causing bowel obstruction and more often ureteral obstruction. The cause of death is typically uremia, due to bilateral ureteral obstruction. The major components of the disease remain local throughout the entire terminal course. Slightly more than one-third of advanced colon cancer patients are in the local pattern.

Hepatic Pattern

The hepatic pattern is characterized by progressive liver involvement due to metastatic deposits (Fig. 2). The early form of the disease is characteristically found in an

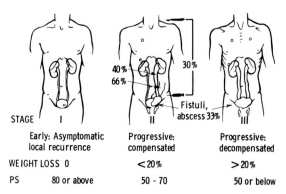

Figure 1. Advanced carcinoma of the large bowel, local pattern. Disease progressive in pelvis, clinically absent or indolent in other areas.

unpredictable form at initial laparotomy. The disease progresses to cause enlargement and discomfort. This leads to eventual liver failure and death. Typically, although the patient may have disease other than in the liver, it is the liver metastasis that causes the major symptoms and kills the patient. The hepatic pattern accounts for about 30% of patients with advanced disease.

Intraabdominal Pattern

The intraabdominal pattern represents transcoelomic spread with multiple metastatic deposits on any peritoneal surfaces (Fig. 3). The pattern also includes omental deposits, and when the peritoneal disease coalesces it forms a rectal shelf and large intraabdominal masses. The mode of spread is reminiscent of ovarian cancer. The progress of the disease includes the development of ascites. Multiple areas of small bowel obstruction lead to death from inanition. Often the entire peritoneal cavity is involved with

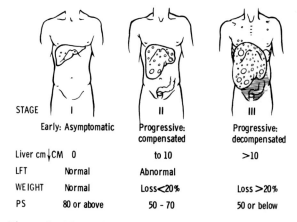

Figure 2. Advanced carcinoma of the large bowel, hepatic pattern. Disease progressive in liver while clinically absent or indolent in other areas.

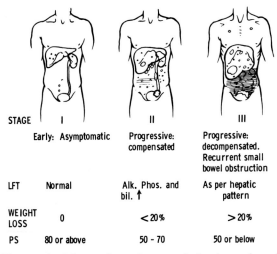

STAGE	I	II	III
	Early: Asymptomatic	Progressive: compensated	Progressive: decompensated. Recurrent small bowel obstruction
LFT	Normal	Alk. Phos. and bil. ↑	As per hepatic pattern
WEIGHT LOSS	0	< 20%	> 20%
PS	80 or above	50 - 70	50 or below

Figure 3. Advanced carcinoma of the large bowel, intraabdominal pattern. Disease progressive within the abdomen and its viscera, but absent or indolent in other areas.

marked reduction in small bowel function. The intraabdominal pattern represents about 14% of the advanced colon cancer population.

Generalized Disease Pattern

The fourth pattern is the generalized disease pattern, which means systemic metastatic cancer (Fig. 4). This includes all areas of distant metastasis, including bone and brain. Lung metastasis, however, is the typical finding. There may be other disease present, such as in the pelvis or liver, but the systemic disease manifesting in the lung or brain is the main problem and is the cause of death. The generalized pattern represents about 20% of advanced colon cancer patients.

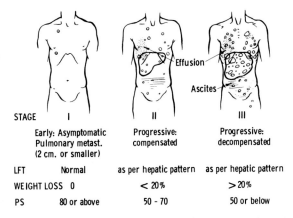

STAGE	I	II	III
	Early: Asymptomatic Pulmonary metast. (2 cm. or smaller)	Progressive: compensated	Progressive: decompensated
LFT	Normal	as per hepatic pattern	as per hepatic pattern
WEIGHT LOSS	0	< 20%	> 20%
PS	80 or above	50 - 70	50 or below

Figure 4. Advanced carcinoma of the large bowel, generalized pattern. Disease progressive generally.

Performance Status

The second element of our calssification is based on the Karnofsky performance status (Fig. 5). This is a clinical evaluation of the percentage functional ability of the patient to perform according to normal activity and status. Thus, 100% is a completely well state; the patient is without symptoms and able to perform usual work. Zero percent is death. The resulting clinical performance rating yields a very practical and essential mark to the progress of disease or the results of treatment. Thus an individual patient, at any given time of the history of his or her disease, can be defined as functioning at a given percentage of normal. This basic classification leads to a further subdivision that is helpful for an understanding of advanced colon cancer. A performance status in the upper third, 80% or better of normal activity, is referred to as Stage-I disease. Patients in Stage I are basically asymptomatic and their disease is stable. A performance status of 40 to 80%, the middle third of the scale, is referred to as Stage-II disease. The cancer in this stage is progressive and only partially compensated; a reduction in activity is necessary as the symptoms increase. The end of the scale, the bottom third, implies a performance status of less than 40% in Stage-III disease, or uncompensated progressive cancer. This represents a preterminal state. Patients in Stage III are candidates for symptomatic relief of their disease and are not subjected to treatments other than for relief of pain. Other therapeutic agents do not contribute to these patients and may add to their burden.

The advantage of these two systemic classifications is apparent when they are combined (Fig. 6). There are four patterns and three stages of advanced colon cancer. The result is a classification that can categorize any patient at any point in his or her disease. This allows the physician to assess effectiveness of treatment and to compare with other

	%	
Able to carry on normal activity; no special care is needed.	100	Normal; no complaints; no evidence of disease.
	90	Able to carry on normal activity; minor signs or symptoms of disease.
	80	Normal activity with effort; some signs or symptoms of disease.
Unable to work; able to live at home; cares for most personal needs; a varying amount of assistance is needed.	70	Cares for self; unable to carry on normal activity or to do active work.
	60	Requires occasional assistance but is able to care for most of his needs.
	50	Requires considerable assistance and frequent medical care.
Unable to care for self; requires equivalent of institutional or hospital care; disease may be progressing rapidly.	40	Disabled; requires special medical care and assistance.
	30	Severely disabled; hospitalization is indicated, although death not imminent.
	20	Very sick; hospitalization necessary; active supportive treatment necessary.
	10	Moribund; fatal processes progressing rapidly.
	0	Dead.

Figure 5. Criteria of performance status (PS).

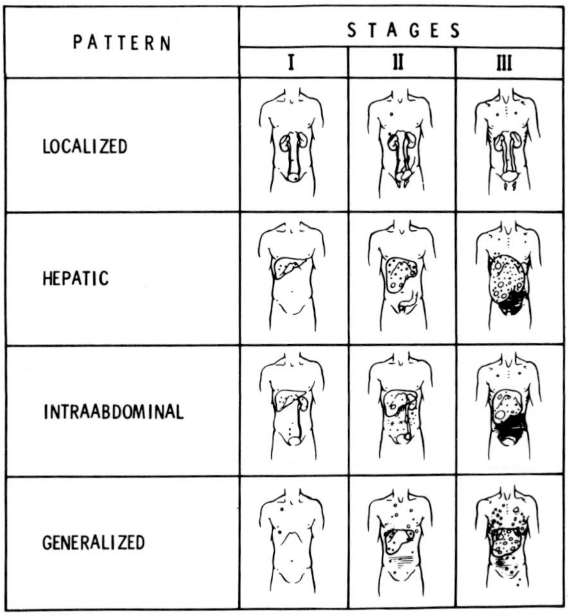

Figure 6. Large bowel carcinoma; the four patterns. Composite of two classifications.

patients in the same category. Hopefully, the adoption of a classification such as this will end the averaging of results from patients with early liver disease and those of patients with terminal carcinomatosis to arrive at treatment protocols. The theoretical hope is that patients will be categorized and then a treatment schedule for this group developed. There is some progress already in this manner. The stage-II local pattern characterized by symptomatic pelvic disease is now treated by pelvic radiation therapy of 3,000 to 4,000 rads with an expected symptomatic response of 80%. As previously mentioned, all Stage-III disease is excluded from treatment schedules except for symptomatic relief or experimental protocols.

BASIC DATA IN ADVANCED COLON CANCER

To establish basic data for advanced colon cancer all patients seen by the Rectum and Colon Service satisfying this classification from the three years 1971–1973 were categorized and followed for five years. All patients were followed. The classification and categorizing was done prospectively and by a single observer. The patients were subjected to all forms of therapy available at that time. This included radiation and chemotherapy, both regular and experimental. There were patients who received no treatment. In this group there was no attempt to compare methods of treatment because of the small numbers involved. Instead the numbers and results reflect basic data in length of survival for the individual patterns and stages. It is suggested that more current methods of treatment be compared with this basic data to indicate advances in clinical therapy, if any.

Table 2. Advanced Colon and Rectum Cancer:
Classification of 267 Patients

	Stage		
Pattern	I	II	III
Localized	11	85	1
97 36%			
Hepatic	24	52	2
78 30%			
Intraabdominal	10	25	3
38 14%			
Generalized	3	47	4
54 20%			

Two hundred sixty-seven patients were seen, categorized, and followed in the time period 1971–1973. The patients were placed by pattern and stage (Table 2). All patients were included. There were no exclusions or exceptions. In the local pattern there were 97 patients, or 36% of the total. Within this pattern 11 were stage I, 85 were stage II, and 1 was stage III. In the hepatic pattern there were 78 patients, or 30% of the total, divided into 24 in Stage I, 52 in Stage II, and 2 in stage III. The intraabdominal pattern included 38 patients, or 14% of the total, with 10 in Stage I, 25 in Stage II, and 3 in Stage III. Finally, the generalized disease pattern accounted for 54 patients, or 20% of the total, with 3 in Stage I, 47 in Stage II, and 4 in Stage III.

All 267 patients were followed to death or for a minimum of 5 years. The survival data provide a definite baseline for future studies as well as a definite reflection of the natural history of advanced large-bowel cancer (Table 3). Thus, of the 267 patients, 177 died the first year, leaving 90, or 34%. An additional 57 died the second year, leaving 33, or 12%. At the end of 36 months, an additional 30 had succumbed to their disease, leaving 13 or 5%. At the end of five years all but four patients were dead. The five-year survival for advanced colon cancer is 1.5%.

The figures can be arranged by pattern to indicate percentage of survival (Table 4). In the local pattern the one-year survival is 44%, while it is 31% in the hepatic pattern group. The intraabdominal and generalized one-year survival were even less, at 21% and 28%. At the two-year period 20% of local-pattern patients were alive against 10% or less of the other patterns. The remainder of the data are proportionate, but the numbers of patients surviving are quite small by three years. The local pattern does have a

Table 3. Advanced Colon and Rectum Cancer:
Survival Data for 267 Patients

	1 yr	2 yr	3 yr	5 yr
Number survivors	90	33	13	4
Percentage survivors	34%	12%	5%	1.5%

Table 4. Advanced Colon and Rectum Cancer:
Survival by Pattern

	<1 yr	<2 yr	<3 yr	+5 yr
Localized	44%	20%	7%	4%
Hepatic	31%	10%	3%	0%
Intraabdominal	21%	8%	5%	0%
Generalized	28%	5%	4%	0%

better prognosis in comparison with the other patterns; the four patients to survive five years were all local pattern. No patient in any of the other patterns lived five years. Thus a patient with liver metastasis has only a 3% chance of surviving three years and none of living five years. There may be an occasional exception, but none were recorded here. Similar interpretations can be made for the other patterns, which include the lung metastasis in the generalized pattern, where 4% lived three years and again no patients survived five years. A further interpretation of the material may aid the clinician in interpreting individual survival profiles.

In each pattern and stage a determination can be made of the time in months when 50% of the patients in that group had expired. These data have more meaning than the average survival (Table 5). In the local pattern one-half of the patients in the asymptomatic or Stage-I group were dead within 11 months. In the Stage-II symptomatic group one-half were dead within 10 months. As would be expected the 50% survival in Stage-III disease was very short in all patterns. Of the patients with asymptomatic liver metastasis one-half will be dead in 12 months, while if the measure is taken when symptoms are discernible, the 50% survival is only 7 1/2 months. In the intraabdominal-pattern half of the patients with peritoneal seeding, those with Stage-I disease will be dead in nine months, while with symptomatic clinical abdominal carcinomatosis half will be dead in three months. Similarly the generalized-disease pattern half of the asymptomatic patients with lung metastasis will be dead in 12 1/2 months, while when the measure is taken with onset of clinical symptoms, half will be dead in seven months.

In another interpretation, for a given treatment to be meaningful in a given population group with symptomatic liver metastasis, one-half of the patients would have to sur-

Table 5. Advanced Colon and Rectum Cancer:
50% Survival in Months

		Stage	
Pattern	*I*	*II*	*III*
Localized 11 months	11	10	1
Hepatic 8 months	12	7.5	1
Intraabdominal 4 months	9	3	1
Generalized 7 months	12.5	7	3

vive over 7 1/2 months. This precludes an unselected patient population as has been done here. These data also allow for an interpretation to account for the occasional patient who may live four years with advanced disease. Considerable care has to be exercised in interpreting this survival time as a result of therapy as it may only be the true natural history of the stage and pattern. The intention here is to stimulate an interest in the concerned clinician to concentrate thinking on a particular unfortunate group of patients with advanced disease and attempting by the tools at hand to improve these dismal results.

OTHER MANAGEMENT CONSIDERATIONS

Pain

Pain in advanced cancer is a major problem and demands control. It is striking that even though the progress of the disease is pronounced, relatively small amounts of medication judiciously administered can control pain. Aspirin and aspirinlike drugs are efficient in the early stages, while codeine derivatives are helpful later. Large doses of morphine are rarely needed in colon cancer. Even when more potent narcotics are necessary frequent small doses of Levo-Dromoran and methadone are quite efficient. The effective use of medication aids the family in caring for an individual with minimal sedation. Analgesics are constipating and small doses of laxative such as milk of magnesia used frequently can obviate distressing constipation; 30- to 60-cc daily doses, depending on the amount of analgesics taken, can be very helpful. This is true even in the presence of a colostomy. The relief of symptoms of constipation may offer the patient considerable relief from abdominal and pelvic pressure.

Occasionally, more severe pelvic and perineal pain may not be relieved by medication or radiation therapy. In patients where bowel and bladder control is less of a factor, permanent saddle-block anesthesia with intrathecal alcohol can be effective. This is performed by the anesthesiologist. Neurosurgical procedures such as cordotomy and other central-nerve interruption procedures are offered infrequently and rarely accepted by our patients. The described complications of these procedures outweigh the anticipated relief of pain. There have been no patients who accepted a major neurosurgical procedure for relief of pain on the Rectum and Colon Service for over 10 years.

Nutrition

The nutritional aspects of advanced cancer are important. The use of techniques that force feed or provide parenteral nutrition to prolong life when all reasonable methods of palliation have been exhausted is to be condemned. The use of these techniques can be helpful to restore nutrition before and after surgery for obstruction when bowel continuity has been reestablished.

Perineal Disease

The patient with advanced cancer in the perineum, which is ulcerated, infected, and fungating, presents a major unsolvable problem. This is particularly true when radiation therapy and chemotherapy are no longer effective. This is one of the most distressing problems in advanced rectal cancer. Patients and their families are distressed by the odor and the persistent bleeding from the fungating mass. There is no completely satisfactory answer. Perineal irrigations of dilute permanganate solution can reduce infection and drainage. Fulguration techniques to cauterize and remove volume may help but are often bloody. Cryosurgical techniques with deep-probe freezing has produced nonhemorrhagic sloughs effecting removal of tumor bulk and has made patient acceptance and nursing care less trying. This major problem offers a challenge to the managing physician.

SUMMARY

Consideration of the possibility of surgical resection of advanced disease is primary before further therapy is instituted. The absolute documentation of nonresectability must be established as an initial concept. Opportunities for surgical palliation must be considered. This is particularly important in bowel obstruction and large abdominal masses.

Nonresectable advanced cancer of the colon and rectum can be classified into stage and pattern. Use of this schemata can add to the specific care and management of the individual patient. The reporting of results of current and new therapy would benefit by use of this method.

The overall survival rate of patients with advanced cancer of the large bowel is most disheartening. The three-year survival rate is less than 5%. The informed and concerned practitioner who has an understanding of the scope of the problem and is interested in the management of these patients offers the best palliation currently available.

REFERENCE

1. Young C, Ellison R, Sullivan R, et al.: Evaluation of therapeutic response of large bowel cancer to the fluorinated pyrimidenes in relation to clinical patterns (abstract). *Proc Am Assn Cancer Res* 3:164, 1960.

9

Uncommon
Malignant Anal
and Rectal Tumors

Stuart H. Q. Quan

GENERAL COMMENTS

At the outset, in any discussion of anal and rectal tumors, it is important to stress the obvious; namely, that a correct diagnosis is based on a high index of suspicion on the part of the examining physician, who then provides adequate biopsy material so that the pathologist can arrive at the true histologic diagnosis.

Leukoplakia (Fig. 1), chronic hemorrhoids, anal fissure, lymphogranuloma venereal, chronic fistulas, and previously irradiated anal skin and anal condylomas (Fig. 2) have all been considered as potential predisposing causes in the development of cancer of the anal area (particularly squamous carcinoma of the anorectum). Although we are uncertain that there is an etiologic relationship, we must not be misled by these conditions into ruling out a possible underlying cancer.

Symptoms produced by an anal neoplasm, regardless of histologic type, are no different from those seen with more common inflammatory and nonmalignant conditions; such symptoms are usually nonspecific. A patient with either condition can describe pruritus, burning, pain, discomfort, bleeding, drainage, sensation of a mass, and so on. These common complaints, if considered trivial by the patient and physician, can delay an early diagnosis of a malignant tumor in the anal region.

In order of ascending frequency of occurrence, the following malignant tumors of the anal canal and anal margin will be discussed: basal cell carcinoma, extramammary Paget's disease, Bowen's disease or in situ epidermoid carcinoma, malignant melanoma, and epidermoid carcinoma (invasive). Leiomyoma and leiomyosarcoma, malignant lymphomas, and carcinoid tumors of the rectum and colon, will be described separately. Acute anorectal complications in leukemic patients will also be considered. It is worthwhile to mention in passing that at MSKCC, we have also seen in a few instances adenocarcinoma of the rectum that had grown out of the rectum to occupy the anal and perianal area (Fig. 3), but this is extremely rare.

The relative rarity of these tumors in the anus and rectum can be brought into perspective by comparing the number of these lesions to the total number of malignant tumors seen in this same anatomic area at the Memorial Sloan-Kettering Cancer Center

115

from 1929 through 1974, a span of 45 years. Approximately 400 of these uncommon neoplasms are herein described against a backdrop of almost 10,000 malignant tumors of the distal intestinal tract; this represents an incidence of 4%. By far the most common of these uncommon lesions is epidermoid cancer of the anorectum, which comprises three-fourths of this group of rare tumors (Fig. 4).

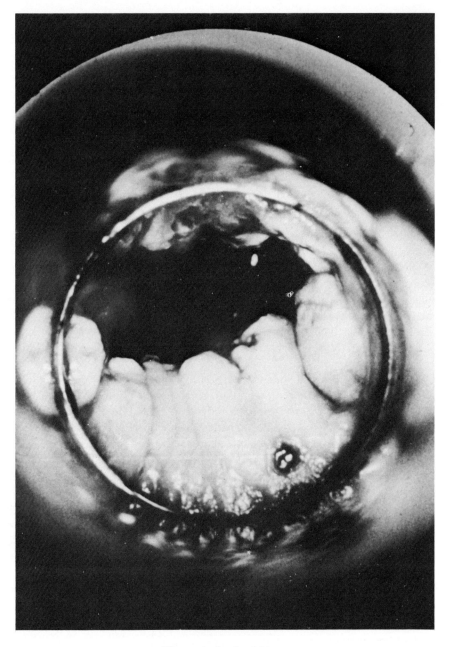

Figure 1. Leukoplakia.

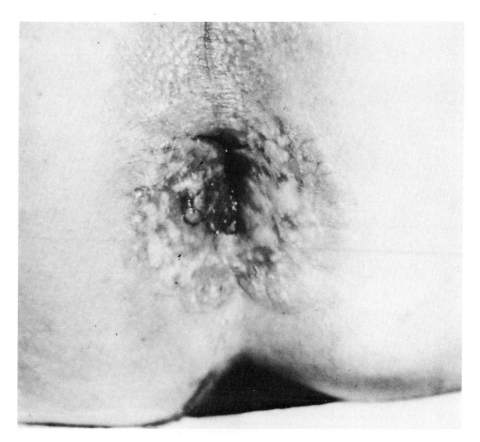

Figure 2. Condylomas.

BASAL CELL CARCINOMA

Basal cell carcinoma (Fig. 5), or rodent ulcer of the anal margin, is an extremely unusual tumor. The St. Mark's Hospital experience reports only 10 such lesions in this anatomic area in over 4,000 malignant tumors (1), and at Memorial Hospital, only five such patients are so listed in the past 25 years. These were three men and two women, whose average age was in the late fifties. Characteristically, the tumor has distinct rolled edges, with a central shallow ulceration, and has never been described to invade deeper or adjacent structures, or to metastasize.

Histologically the picture is that of an epithelial tumor arising from the basal cells of the malpighian layer of the skin. It is made up of compact sheets of basophilic staining cells containing large blue-staining nuclei with minimal cytoplasm.

Adequate surgical excision virtually assures a cure. Primary closure is usually possible if the tumor is small, and partial closure leaving the rest of the wound to heal by secondary intention if the tumor is large, is rarely necessary.

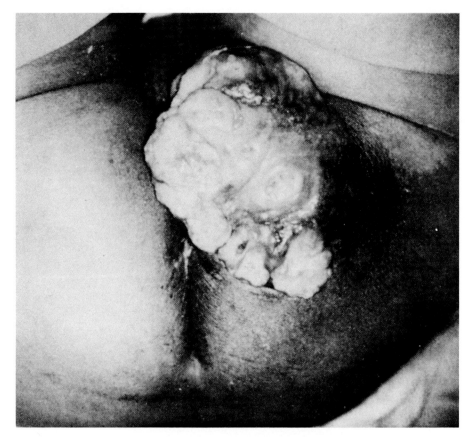

Figure 3. Adenocarcinoma from rectum invading perianal region.

PERIANAL PAGET'S DISEASE

Perianal Paget's disease, or extramammary Paget's disease, of the perianal region, since its first description in 1949 by Foraker (2), represents an unusually rare clinicopathological entity. Arminski and Pollard in a review in 1973 can cite only 32 reported cases from the medical literature (3) . Since our original study of 1975 reporting seven patients, we have seen only two other patients with this disease (4).

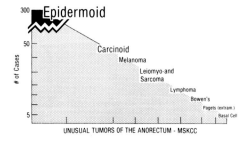

Figure 4. Unusual tumors of the anorectum.

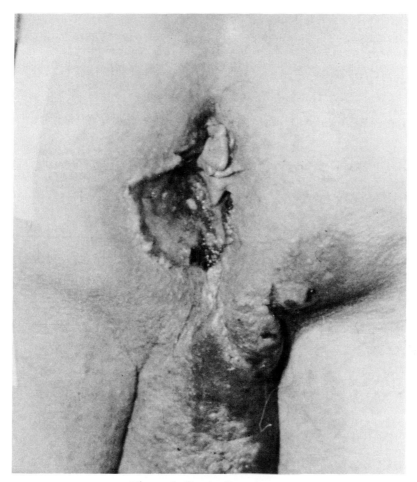

Figure 5. Basal-cell carcinoma.

Clinical Features

Our patients vary in age from 46 to 69 years, with a mean of about 58. There were five males and four females afflicted. The presenting symptoms were usually nonspecific but sufficient to draw attention to the anatomic region for biopsy with resultant histologic diagnosis. The clinical dermatologic manifestation is that of a pale grey, crusty, plaque-like lesion (Figs. 6, 7) that may be indurated and/or inflamed. Those lesions with an underlying cancer often present as a mass, and three of our patients already had inguinal metastases when they were first seen by us. Three other patients, who had long-standing complaints, also had the most confluent superficial skin changes without an underlying carcinoma.

Pathologic diagnosis resulted from detection of large, single, pale intraepithelial cells as a prominent histologic feature, whose cytoplasm stained positively with the aldehyde-fuchsin stain. These cells distinguished this condition from other entities such as Bowen's disease and/or malignant melanoma. Indeed, in three of our nine patients the diagnostic confusion between Bowen's and Paget's existed initially, until further stain studies differentiated the two. Unlike the Paget's disease of the nipple, which almost always overlies a mammary-duct carcinoma, extramammary Paget's disease may not necessarily be associated with an invasive tumor. Thus, subjacent infiltrating carcinoma, usually colloid in type, was found in five of nine of our patients. All these cancers were thought to arise from a perianal gland or other skin appendage, and not from the rectal mucosa.

Treatment and Prognosis

Treatment and prognosis depend, of course, on the presence or absence of an underlying invasive carcinoma. If present, treatment is directed toward the underlying carcinoma with complete surgical eradication. If invasive carcinoma is not present, local excision with clear margins is sufficient. Our patients who had Paget's disease of the anus without underlying invasive carcinoma were cured, although multiple excisions were required. All the patients who had perianal Paget's disease with invasive carcinoma that had already metastasized to the inguinal nodes did poorly and died, despite surgical treatment as well as x-ray therapy and 5-fluorouracil chemotherapy. When extramammary Paget's disease was associated with early localized invasive carcinoma, as we had in one patient, wide local excisions were sufficient to cure the patient, who is now alive, 17 years after original discovery of his disease, even though recurrent adenocarcinoma

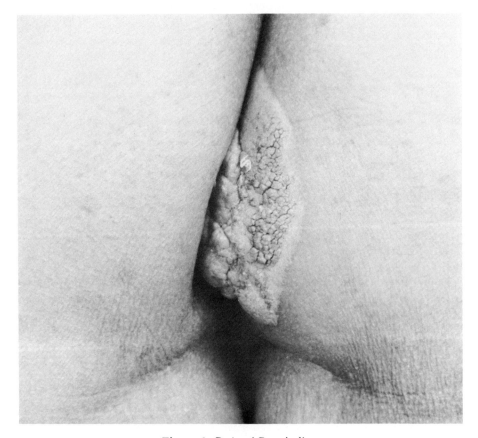

Figure 6. Perianal Paget's disease.

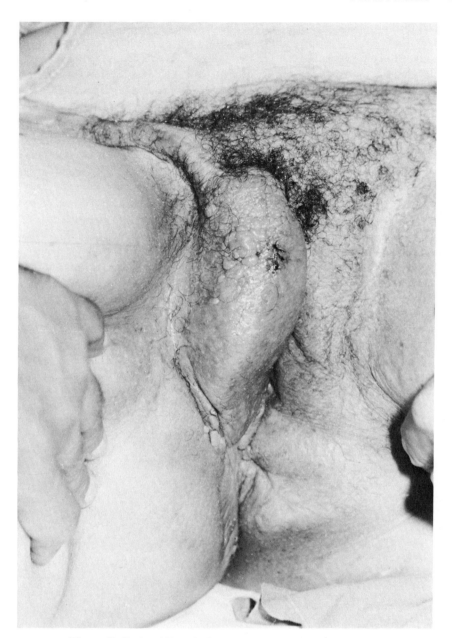

Figure 7. Perianal Paget's disease recurrent in the labia majora.

was found six and 12 years after the original excision. The recurrence was excised on each occasion.

BOWEN'S DISEASE

Bowen's disease is a chronic intraepithelial squamous-cell carcinoma first described by Dr. John Bowen in 1912 (5). It is better known to dermatologists, who more commonly see it on the face, hands, and trunk, than it is to other specialists. Rarely does it occur in the genital area, and according to the literature even more rarely in the perianal area. Fewer than 100 patients have been reported to have Bowen's disease in this area (8). The specific clinical implication of this dermatologic curiosity is its association with simultaneous or subsequent development of other cancers in the same patient.

Clinically it appears as a discrete, reddish, plaquelike area, with scaly looking eczematoid features (Fig. 8). The differential diagnosis of Bowen's disease includes basal cell carcinoma, solar keratosis, and extramammary Paget's disease. The histologic picture is that of an in situ squamous carcinoma confined to the epidermis. There is striking loss of normal cell progression with marked hyperkeratosis, parakeratosis, plaquelike acanthosis, and inflammatory infiltrate. The Bowenoid cells frequently have large hyperchromatic nuclei with some vacuolization to give them a haloed effect. In contrast to Paget's disease, a Bowenoid cell does not pick up aldehyde-fuchsin stain.

We have seen 12 patients with this disease at Memorial Hospital up to 1977 (6). These were seven women and five men, and the ages vary from 32 to 74, with a mean age of 54. One patient subsequently developed focally invasive epidermoid carcinoma in the anal margin; one had concomitant Bowen's disease of the vulva, carcinoma in situ of the cervix, and hamartoma of the liver; and two other patients had coexistent cancer of the colon. Primary choice of treatment is wide local full-thickness excision with additional resection of the margins for frozen section to insure adequate removal. Effective responses to the topical application of 5-fluorouracil and dinitrochlorobenzene ointment have also been recently reported (7).

Five of our patients were living and well without disease 5 to 24 years following surgical treatment. One died of a concomitant cancer of the colon 4½ years after discovery,

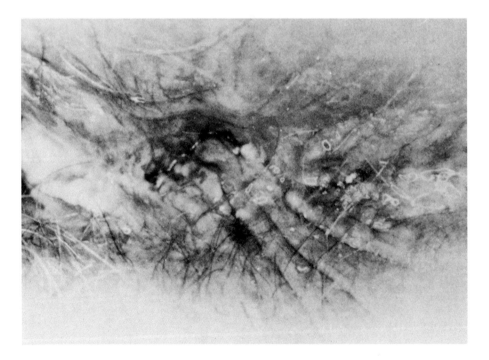

Figure 8. Bowen's disease.

and one is living with disease two years after treatment. The remaining patients are currently still being studied, one with and two without disease less than two years after treatment.

MALIGNANT MELANOMA

Of all the uncommon malignant tumors of the anal area to describe, the most discouraging is malignant melanoma of the anorectum, because of its poor prognosis following surgical treatment (9–13,15). This is in turn due to the fact that, unlike malignant melanoma elsewhere on the skin of the body, which is much more discernible to the patient, and usually receives earlier treatment, this tumor, occurring in an obscure area, the anal canal, most often remains undetected until it causes symptoms. By this time, the tumor is advanced to the histologic "levels of invasion" and has become quite thick, with resultant poor prognosis (16).

A small consolation is the relative rarity of this tumor. From 1929 to 1975 only 49 patients with this disease represent our total experience at the Memorial Sloan-Kettering Cancer Center (14). Approximately 200 such patients have been reported in the medical literature.

Clinical Features

Among our patients, the youngest was 21 and the oldest 85 years of age. The mean and average age was about 58. There were 27 women and 22 men; except for one black woman, and one other woman who was half black and half Chinese, all the patients were white Caucasian. Because most of these tumors arose from or very near the anoderm, the majority of the patients had the sensation of an abnormal mass present. These were usually believed to be hemorrhoids or polyps until the true nature of the lesion was determined by histologic examination. In addition to the feeling of the mass, rectal bleeding was the next most common complaint. The bleeding was usually minor, but steady or recurrent, and not unlike that seen in patients with bleeding hemorrhoids. Pain was not a prominent symptom, and apparently several of the patients experienced little or no disability in this area at all. The duration of symptoms before diagnosis and treatment did not appear to have any influence on the ultimate survival time of the patients. Metastatic inguinal lymphadenopathy was present in seven of our patients, and neurologic changes were prominent in one patient. In each of these patients only careful search revealed the site of the primary lesion to be in the anorectum, and all these patients died within months after the diagnosis of malignant melanoma was made.

The primary tumor varied in appearance from that of a small, benign-looking, grape-like growth at the mucocutaneous junction to that of a large, ulcerating, deeply pigmented tumor occluding the anus (Figs. 9, 10). Melanomas that are considered early are usually flat and superficial, whereas nodularity indicates advanced disease. Thus, the gross pathologic features in our series of patients all indicate how long the disease has been present. Only 13 of our patients had a mass less than 1 cm in size. The remainder measured up to 6 cm in diameter with 4 cm as an average size.

Pigmentation was sufficiently significant to be visible to the unaided eye in over half of the patients, varying from a light grey to a violaceous black color. In the remaining patients pigmentation was observed microscopically only, or pigmentation was absent in a small number, whose disease was diagnosed histologically as amelanotic melanoma.

Histology

The morphologic characteristics of these anorectal melanomas differed in no way from those seen elsewhere in the body. The cells of the various tumors varied atypically from marked spindle to polyhedral shaped, many having a triangular outline. In some cases pleomorphism was marked and the cell border typically well outlined. The cytoplasm, while generally abundant, showed no constant characteristic. The appearance of the nuclei varied; intranuclear vacuoles were seen and multinucleated cells as well were found in many cases. The arrangement of the cells varied from the typical so-called alveolar pattern, where the cells were grouped in nest-like configurations, to a diffuse haphazard distribution throughout the tumor. Mitoses varied markedly in number from case to case.

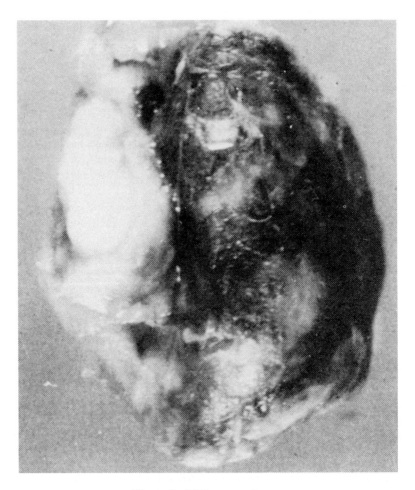

Figure 9. Malignant melanoma.

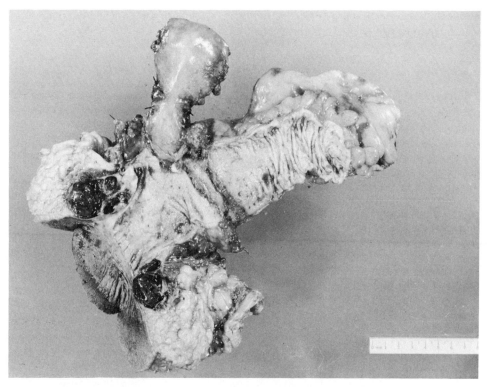

Figure 10. Malignant melanoma of the anorectum (exenteration specimen).

Treatment and Prognosis

Although there have been isolated reported instances in the medical literature of long-term survivors following mere local excision of malignant melanoma of the anus, closer observation of these reports indicate that these tumors where very small and unsuspected, and were discovered only after routine examination of tissue removed at hemorrhoidectomy. Unfortunately, these are very rare occurrences. In our series of patients, covering a period of over 50 years, utilizing procedures ranging from local excisions to abdominoperineal resections with pelvic lymph-node dissection as well, the few good results we have had have only come with radical surgery. Thus, only five of our patients have lived beyond the five-year survival mark following abdominoperineal resection for this disease. This small number again points to the unusually advanced state of the tumor at the time of discovery and diagnosis.

Current studies using different chemotherapeutic as well as immunologically stimulating agents in conjunction with and or without autologous vaccine in the treatment of malignant melanoma of the skin are on trial, but no specific beneficial effect on the treatment of malignant melanoma of the anorectum has been described.

EPIDERMOID CARCINOMA

Epidermoid or squamous carcinoma of the anus is an interesting lesion for study because of its frequent occurrence relative to the less common malignant tumors of the same anatomic area described above (18). The threat it can pose to the patient's life is offset by early diagnosis and proper treatment.

Incidence

Although it may represent 3.9% of all cancers arising in the distal 18 cm of the intestinal tract, if only the perianal, anal, and distal 2 cm of the intestinal tracts are considered, it constitutes 30% of all malignant anal tumors (24). Our continued interest in periodic evaluation and management of this lesion now includes the records of over 300 such patients seen in our institution up to 1975, and we have come to formulate certain criteria that have guided us in the diagnosis and treatment of this particular lesion.

Clinical Features

The average age of our patients was 58; the youngest patient was 22 and the oldest 88 years of age. Females outnumbered males 2 to 1. Symptoms of bleeding, distress, change of intestinal habits or sensation of a mass continue to dominate in frequency of complaints mentioned by the patients. Thus, 136 patients described bleeding as an initial symptom. Seventy-five patients complained of constipation, while 30 had diarrhea. Twenty-seven patients were aware of a lump, and most complained of distress or pain in the anal region. Miscellaneous complaints consisted of excessive flatus, tenesmus, soilage, perianal itch, and so on.

The clinical appearance of epidermoid cancer of the anorectum depends on the state and location of the tumor and may be manifest in a variety of pictures. If the lesion is discovered early, it may appear as a superficial warty growth at the anal margin. As it grows larger and infiltrates the anal canal (Fig. 11), underlying induration and ulceration can be palpated. Further encroachment of the canal can produce scallapoid folds of tumor tissue surrounding the anal opening with spread of the disease via the dermal lymphatics to form satellite nodules along the skin of the groin (Fig. 12). More peripheral tumors can occupy the perianal skin without invasion into the anorectum (Fig. 13).

Because of its anatomic location, inguinal metastasis is not an uncommon occurrence (Fig. 14), and therefore the groin regions should always be carefully palpated in patients with epidermoid cancer of the anal region. To reemphasize: to arrive at a correct diagnosis and subsequent proper management, the physician should follow up any suspicious symptoms with a careful digital and proctoscopic examination. The exact location and size of the tumor in its relation to the dentate line or pectinate line of the anorectum, and its depth of invasion into the subcutaneous tissue, into the musculature, or into the submucosa of the rectum, was to be determined. Adequate tissue biopsy may require the administration of local or general anesthesia.

In describing the histologic diagnosis, the pathologist may use terms such as transitional, cloacogenic, basaloid, basosquamous, or mucoepidermoid types of squamous carcinoma. These multicellular types only reflect the multicytologic origin of the anorectum, and although they present a fascinating and varied histologic picture to the pathologist, as far as the surgeon is concerned in clinical management of the disease, these histologic diagnoses can all be considered as variants of squamous carcinoma in the anal region.

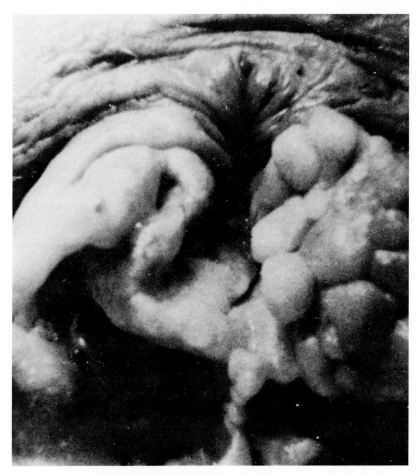

Figure 11. Epidermoid carcinoma, anus.

Treatment

The treatment of this tumor is surgical, and it is emphatic that this is dependent on a careful evaluation of its anatomic location. Those tumors occurring superficially at or below the dentate line, for example, in the lower half of the anal canal or perianal tissues, and are superficial, small, and/or moveable, can be locally but widely excised. The margins of the skin tissues are carefully examined for microscopic evidence of tumor, to ensure complete excision.

The larger lesions that show infiltration into the sphincter or underlying tissues should receive a Miles type of resection with a wide perianal phase of excision, to include as much of the levator muscles as possible as well as the contents of the ischiorectal fossae. Whereas large infiltrating perianal lesions can metastasize along the perianal lymphatics to the scrotum and inguinal nodes, the penetrating ones at the dentate-line junction may in addition spread upward to the mesenteric lymph nodes and/or laterally along the levator muscles to the obturator, iliac, and other extramesenteric pelvic lymph nodes.

Tumors arising above the dentate line and involving the rectum certainly deserve a

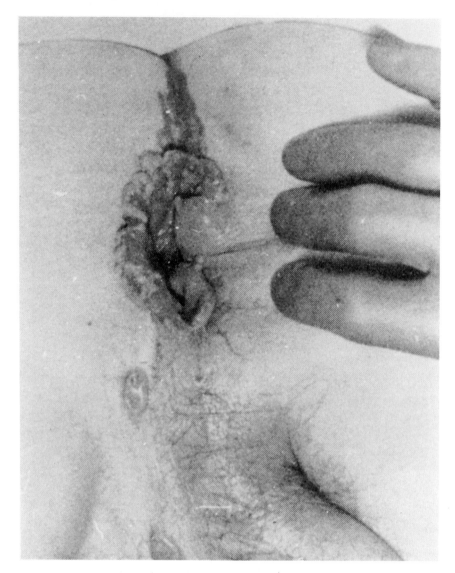

Figure 12. Epidermoid carcinoma with lymphatic satellitosis.

Miles type resection with a wide perineal phase of excision. The treatment of a tumor that has penetrated into the rectovaginal septum of a woman involves at least an inclusive posterior, if not subtotal, vaginectomy. In men, where either prostate, base of bladder, or seminal vesicles are involved, a pelvic exenteration, including cystectomy and construction of an ileobladder, might be indicated. For these deeper lesions, and if the patient is a good surgical risk, additional pelvic lymph-node dissection may be included in the abdominoperineal resection phase of the operation.

The lymph nodes in the inguinal regions, unless histologically proved to be positive for metastasis, are untreated (25). Based on our statistical analysis (22,23), a therapeutic rather than a prophylactic groin dissection is recommended. The simultaneous appearance of inguinal metastasis and an untreated primary tumor in a patient is an ominous sign. Very few of these patients, despite radical surgery, live five years after discovery of the disease. On the other hand, in those patients whose inguinal metastasis appears subsequent to treatment of their primary tumor, and who then receive groin dissection, the prognosis is much better, because the majority of them are alive and well at the five-year level (24). That is why strict periodic surveillance of the inguinal region following initial surgery for the primary lesion is mandatory.

We have steered away from x-ray therapy as the treatment of choice for epidermoid carcinoma of the anorectum, although, in selected patients, favorable results have been reported. Multimodality treatment using chemotherapy and radiotherapy for the pelvis before surgery for this disease has also been effective in the management of the tumor (19–21). This represents an ongoing study, in which approximately 21 patients have so been treated. The chemotherapist uses intravenous mitomycin C and 5-fluorouracil (5-FU) in a sequential fashion. The mitomycin is given intravenously in one dose calculated at 15 mg/m^2 of the patient's body. This is followed by a five-day continuous intravenous drip of 5-FU calculated at 750 mg/m^2 of the patient's body. Then radiotherapy to the pelvis to include the perineum of 3,000 rads is given over a period of three weeks. The results are too early to assess, but the immediate and palliative effect can be striking. Eight patients, after favorable response to this protocol, have been sub-

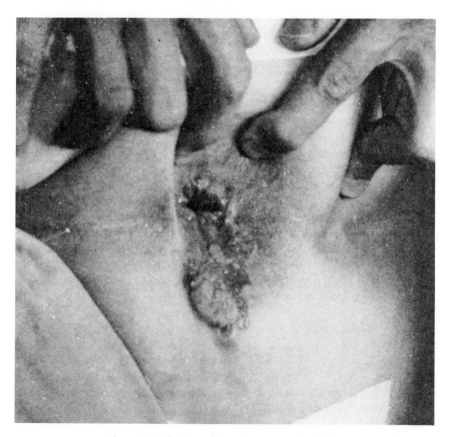

Figure 13. Epidermoid carcinoma, perianal skin.

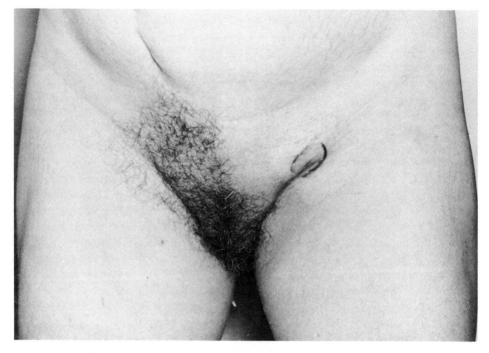

Figure 14. Inguinal metastasis from epidermoid carcinoma anus.

jected to radical surgery, and their resected specimens have shown only microscopic residual or no residual disease at all. Thirteen other patients, whose pretreatment tumors would have required radical surgery, after chemotherapy and radiotherapy required only local excisional surgery. Another five years will have to elapse before we can evaluate the efficacy of this experimental way of treating this particular tumor.

Results

The results of treatment at Memorial Hospital of 299 patients with epidermoid carcinoma of the anus have been divided into three periods as follows: In the series of patients seen between 1944 and 1963, the five-year overall survival rate for 109 patients was 53%, and for those who were treated surgically it was 57% (24). In the series of 125 patients seen prior to 1944, the five-year overall survival rate was only 29% of the total group seen, and 41% for the patients treated surgically (17). This improvement in the survival rate in these two series from the same institution can be attributed to early recognition by the patient, early diagnosis by the physician, and an attempt at proper choice of treatment according to the size of the primary tumor, its location, and potential lymphatic dissemination.

In the most recent series of 65 patients seen between 1964 and 1970, however, the overall five-year survival rate has dropped back to 25%, and only 33% for the patients treated surgically. The analysis of this apparent setback reveals that many of these patients have more advanced disease in their initial examination at our hospital (as illustrated by the fact that only 16 of the 65 patients were considered eligible for local excision alone). This dire retrogression points up again the continued need for patient education and for earlier diagnosis and therapy by the physician.

LEIOMYOMA AND LEIOMYOSARCOMA OF THE RECTUM AND COLON

Smooth-muscle tumors of the gastrointestinal tract occur rarely. They are less frequently seen in the lower intestinal tract than in the stomach and small intestine. Of the 56 patients with leiomyoma and leiomyosarcoma of the colon and rectum on which this study is based, 17 such tumors of the rectum have been previously reported from this institution (30). A more detailed description, particularly of the 39 new patients hitherto unreported, will be the subject of a forthcoming publication (28). The relative rarity of leiomyosarcoma in the colon and rectum is well-documented in the literature. Recent reviews (27,31) indicate only 29 colonic and slightly more than 100 rectal leiomyosarcomas reported in the world's medical literature.

LEIOMYOMA

Twenty patients (12 men and 8 women) at Memorial Sloan-Kettering Cancer Center had leiomyomas of the colon and rectum. (colon, 10; rectum, 10). The youngest patient was 39 and the oldest 91, with a mean and average age of 63 and 62, respectively.

Seven of the patients exhibited symptoms that were minor and unrelated to their leiomyomas, and 13 asymptomatic patients had their tumors detected in an incidental fashion. Three of these were autopsy findings, four were by routine proctosigmoidoscopy, and six were found at operation for some other primary pathology. The leiomyomas were sessile, polypoid, pedunculated, or covered with intact mucosa, and measured from 0.2 to 4 cm. All responded to some form of local excision, either by cautery snare or by cold-knife removal, and yielded excellent results.

Histologic Features

The benign smooth-muscle tumors were orderly and more highly cellular than normal smooth muscle. The nuclei were small, oval, and regular and there was no appreciable mitotic activity. The internuclear eosinophilic material was all myoplasm. This was revealed by a study of specimens prepared with Van Gieson's stain. This finding is in contrast with results obtained by the same stain on the sarcoma specimen.

LEIOMYOSARCOMAS OF THE RECTUM

Age and Sex

In this series of 24 patients, the youngest was 21 years old and the oldest 73. The mean and average ages were 53 and 52, respectively. There were 15 men and 9 woman. The men on the whole seemed to be younger, having an average age of 41 in contrast to 58 for the women.

Clinical Presentation

In the primary group of 17 patients with previously untreated rectal leiomyosarcoma, pain was prominent in 5 and attributable in 4 of these to the immense size of the tumor. The sensation of a mass in the rectum, constipation, and/or bleeding were also described by each of two patients. Indeed these were all late symptoms and boded a poor prognosis. On physical examination, these patients not only had large rectal tumors, but pararectal (Fig. 15) and vaginal extension was described in two patients each, and one

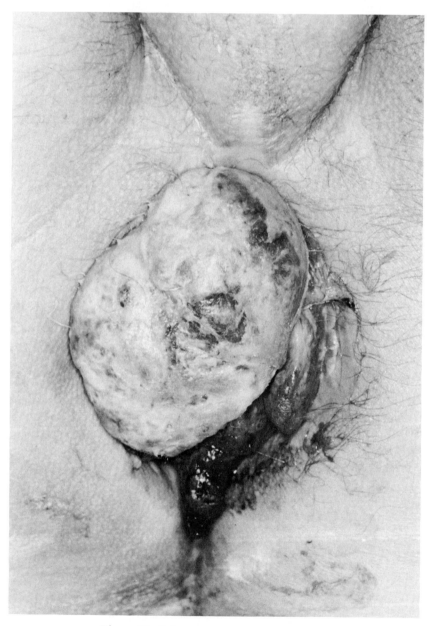

Figure 15. Leiomyosarcoma rectum recurrent.

exhibited a suprapubic mass as well. Fixation and immobility were described in five instances, and the largest tumor was described as big as a fetal head.

Five relatively asymptomatic patients had primary tumors that were picked up on routine proctosigmoidoscopic examination. These tumors were in general much smaller than those of the primary group, they measured from 1 to 2.5 cm in diameter, and were smooth, submucosal, firm, rubbery, hard, or indurated. Ulceration of the overlying rectal mucosa was the exception rather than the rule in the rectal leiomyosarcoma, because of the smooth-muscle origin of the lesion.

Three other patients had a diagnosis of rectal leiomyosarcoma established as a result of surgery performed for another condition. Two men had undergone transurethral resection for prostatic obstruction, and one woman had undergone anorectal fistulectomy, with resultant histologic diagnosis of leiomyosarcoma of the rectum. The malignant-tumor diagnosis was totally unsuspected.

Seven patients who presented with recurrent rectal leiomyosarcoma following treatment elsewhere lacked adequate description of symptoms and physical signs in their records. Pelvic recurrence was described in three, and local rectal, pararectal, and rectal vaginal recurrence was described in each of the remaining patients. Lung metastasis was evident in two patients.

Histologic Features

Variations in the histologic characteristics of leiomyosarcoma were common in our series. Half of the tumors showed enough orderly arrangement to indicate the myomatous origin, varying in transition from this form through loose structure to crowded cellular pleomorphic tumors. Mitosis was common in all tumors, excepting a few, so that there was not the separation between the small low-grade and large high-grade tumors observed by us in examination of gastric leiomyosarcomas (26). Neither cellularity nor the amount of cytoplasm correlated with the size of the tumor or its prognosis. Two of the five smallest leiomyosarcomas were the most pleomorphic, while three of the five largest tumors were less cellular and well-organized. All five small tumors were definitely malignant, as measured by the usual histologic criteria.

Treatment and Results

Five leiomyosarcomas of the rectum were excised locally, and these patients are apparently alive and free of disease when last heard from 11, 12, and 13 years (3 patients), and 16 years (2 patients) after treatment (Table 1). The largest of these tumors measured 2×3 cm and was located in the rectovaginal septum; it yielded to reexcision, following an initial operation for a mistaken diagnosis of rectovaginal fistula.

Of six patients who underwent abdominoperineal resection of the rectum all died of disease in less than five years, except for one, who lived until the sixth year after treatment. Of three patients who underwent pelvic exenteration, one has been living and well eight years, free of disease following radical surgery. The other two died less than two years after pelvic excision.

Two patients, whose disease had extended beyond the confines of the pelvis and therefore were considered inoperable, received radiotherapy and chemotherapy for palliation. One patient lived 11 years before dying of the disease, despite local excision that was followed by immediate proctosigmoidectomy.

Table 1. Five Cases of Leiomyosarcoma Cured by Local Excision

Age, Sex	Symptoms	Location, Size, Gross Appearance of Tumors	Histologic Grading	Treatment	Results	Comments
41 M	None	3 to 4 cm from mucocutaneous junction; encapsulated nodule, 1 cm in diameter	3	Local excision	Living and well 11 years after operation	Cure after local excision only
56 M	Perianal itch associated with prolapsing hemorrhoids; progressive constipation after hemorrhoidectomy	Right rectal wall, 3 cm up; submucosal mass, 1.5 cm in diameter	3	Excision with full thickness of rectal wall	Living and well 16 years after operation	Cure after local excision
60 M	Protrusion of rectal mass	Left anterior wall; mass, 2.5 cm in diameter	3	Cautery-snare excision	Living and well 16 years after operation	Cure after local excision
52 F	Pruritus ani	4 cm or larger; 2 cm in diameter; mucosa adherent; underlying muscularis free	2	Local excision	Living and well 13 years after operation	Cure after local excision
48 F	Painless bleeding, excision of rectovaginal fistula	2 × 3 cm tumor rectovaginal septum		Local excision	Living and well 12 years after operation	Cure after local excision

Of the seven patients who had received their initial treatment elsewhere but whose tumor had recurred, only one patient survived a local recurrence and an abdominoperineal resection for 10 years before succumbing to his disease. The remaining six all died of their disease from 11 months to 4 years after tumor recurrence despite all modes of treatment.

LEIOMYOSARCOMA OF THE COLON

Age and Sex

The age range for the 11 colonic leiomyosarcomas was 18 to 75 with both a median and average age of 57. The sex distribution was almost equal: six men and five women. Again the average age of the men was younger (49 years old) than the women (65 years old).

Clinical Presentation

All but one of the five patients with primary untreated colonic leiomyosarcoma exhibited lower-intestinal symptoms such as bleeding, change in bowel habits, abdominal pain, or weight loss, and so on. Oddly enough, the one asymptomatic patient had a huge right-lower quadrant mass and the largest tumor, measuring 25 × 15 × 10 cm, in the right colon. The smallest tumor measured 6 cm in the sigmoid. All had striking radiographic findings and at least three easily manifested palpable abdominal masses.

Four patients who had invasive disease with either liver or omental or abdominal-wall involvement succumbed to disease within a year after radical en block excision of the colon plus the extracolonic involvement. The patient who had the smallest lesion in the sigmoid (6 cm) lived nine years free of disease and died of another cause. One patient was lost track of and one is still living less than a year without disease, following abdominoperineal resection of the rectum and omentectomy. Three patients whose colonic leiomyosarcoma had been operated on first elsewhere, all died of disease within a year, despite both surgical reexcision and/or chemotherapy and radiotherapy.

In summation, the prognosis and the success or failure in the treatment of patients with colorectal leiomyosarcoma is similar to that of carcinoid (29), in that it is decidedly dependent on the size of the original lesion when first detected. On one hand, five patients with rectal leiomyosarcomas of small size (1–2.5 cm) at the time of their discovery responded to adequate local excision and are long-term survivals; whereas those with the larger tumors, particularly those greater than 6 cm, all did poorly regardless of radical surgery and other adjunctive modalities of treatment.

MALIGNANT LYMPHOMA OF THE COLON AND RECTUM

Malignant lymphoma of the colon and rectum is a rare condition either as a localized entity or as a part of a generalized process (33,35). A recent review of the world's literature yielded fewer than 300 cases (34,36). Up to 1975 we have seen only 28 patients with primary involvement of the colon and rectum by malignant lymphoma, whereas secondary involvement was estimated to be 8% of patients with generalized disease studied in a five-year period. There were 10 patients in whom the primary manifestation of the disease was in the rectal or rectosigmoid area, 8 in the ileocecal segment, 4 in the cecum and ascending colon, and 6 whose disease showed overlapping between rectum, colon, or small bowel. Nineteen of the 28 patients eventually developed generalized lymphoma.

Clinical Features

Seventeen men and eleven women were found in our series of whom 73% were more than 50 years of age. Rectal and/or abdominal mass, pain, and bleeding were the most common clinical signs and symptoms. Whereas diarrhea was more common than constipation, obstructive intestinal symptoms were seen frequently in right-colon disease. In proctosigmoidoscopic examination submucosal involvement was most frequently described, although occasionally the tumor appeared as a polypoid, annular, or diffuse indurated mass. Radiographically, the mass may appear localized or diffuse.

Pathology

Malignant lymphoma may be classified histologically into lymphosarcoma, reticulum cell sarcoma, giant follicular lymphosarcoma, and Hodgkin's disease (32). There were no instances of giant follicular lymphosarcoma or Hodgkin's disease in our series. Three clinical stages are described for the convenience of treatment and results: stage I is localized focus of one anatomic area, stage II is two adjacent anatomic areas on one side of the diaphragm, and stage III indicates generalized disease with multiple-system organ involvement.

Treatment and Results

Generally the treatment was dictated by location, extent, and stage of disease. The three modalities of therapy used were radiation therapy, surgery, and chemotherapy. Radiation therapy was generally used with localized lesions (Stage I) or with symptomatic local areas in the presence of generalized disease (Stage III). Surgery was useful in removing a limited localized area of disease (Stage I). Palliative surgery in generalized or Stage-III disease was also indicated in cases of intestinal obstruction, perforation, intussusception, or intestinal fistula. The five-year survivals were: stage I, 8 of 10 patients; stage II, 4 of 5 patients; and stage III, none.

CARCINOID TUMORS OF THE RECTUM AND COLON

Carcinoid tumors of the rectum and colon are relatively rare. The 41 carcinoid tumors (29 rectal and 12 colonic) on which this report is based represent a hospital experience spanning 26 years, during which time approximately 18,000 other malignant tumors of the large bowel were seen. This represents a mere incidence of 0.002%. Another 39 patients with purely nonmetastasizing rectal carcinoids were seen and treated as outpatients, at the time a cancer-prevention clinic was attached to the hospital unit, where routine proctosigmoidoscopic examinations were done in asymptomatic patients. Both of these series will be updated.

Within the gastrointestinal tract itself, rectal carcinoids were found at least as often if not more so than were carcinoids in the appendix and ileum, because of the practice of routine proctosigmoidoscopy as part of the complete physical examination. In diminishing frequency of occurrence were carcinoids of the colon, stomach, gallbladder, jejunum, and duodenum (41,42).

Age and Sex Distribution

The age range was 23 for the youngest patient and 77 for the oldest, with an overall mean average age of 53. If only the patients with nonmetastasizing rectal carcinoids are considered, their average age was only 48. There was virtually no difference in sex distribution in our series: 39 men and 41 women.

The small, less than 2 cm in diameter, carcinoids that were still intramural in location when detected in the rectum tended not to produce any symptoms. The majority (50/66) of our patients with rectal carcinoids represented this group. The remaining 16 patients with larger tumors usually exhibited serosal invasion and produced symptoms: bleeding, if there was mucosal ulceration, and constipation, on up to pain and intestinal obstruction in the very big lesions. With rare exceptions the colonic carcinoids were symptomatic because of their size, and exhibited invasion to the serosal surface and/or beyond.

Proctosigmoidoscopic Examination

The diagnosis of rectal carcinoids should always be considered when a small, smooth, very firm, sessile submucosal nodule is palpated on examination. The majority of our rectal carcinoids were within 10 cm from the anal verge. On proctosigmoidoscopy, the carcinoid may appear to have a yellowish or orangy hue, appearing paler than an adenomatous polyp. Only the exceptional rectal carcinoid will appear pedunculated. The larger lesion can appear ulcerative, and careful clinical evaluation will usually indicate underlying muscular and/or deeper-tissue invasion.

Successful biopsy required virtually total removal of the small tumor, which in many instances was less than 0.5 cm in diameter. In the case of the bigger tumors, adequate penetration through the mucosa into the lesion was important for obtaining a positive biopsy specimen.

Histology

At first glance, the histologic diagnosis of carcinoid is not always easy. Indeed, an erroneous diagnosis of adenocarcinoma of the rectum or colon was made in a few of our patients, until further microscopic sections for mucin staining were obtained. Despite pseudoglandular structure of the lesion, mucin stains (mucicarmine plus PAS-alcian blue) were consistently negative in the case of carcinoid tumors.

Dr. John Berg of our pathology department has attempted to differentiate histologically between the nonmetastasizing and metastasizing carcinoids, based solely on their microscopic appearance (40), but found this an extremely difficult and risky technique. However, he did come up with new observations that might suggest the more aggressive tumor: ribboning of sheets of tumor cells was less common, and tendency toward formation of larger and more hyperchromatic staining nuclei was more common in the metastasizing carcinoid. Nevertheless, a pathologist is loathe to predict the clinical behavior of a carcinoid on the basis of microscopic section alone. If the terms *benign* and *malignant* have any meaning with regard to carcinoids, they must be based on gross clinical characteristics.

Associated Pathology

Although multiple carcinoids occurring in the small intestine have been reported by us (42) and others (38,39), only two of our patients had two separate carcinoids in their rectums. On the other hand, there was a striking association of other malignant tumors in patients with carcinoids of the lower intestinal tract. Eight patients had simultaneous adenomatous polyps of the rectum, two of whom also had adenocarcinoma of the rectum. Another patient had a rectal cancer with the carcinoid but no adenomatous polyp. One patient each had cancer of the cervix, vulva, and granular-cell myeloblastoma of the cecum. A fourth patient had five primary tumors: cancer of the ovary, carcinoma of the colon, and carcinoid tumor of the rectum simultaneously, and subsequently developed cancer of the breast, as well as a basal-cell cancer of the nose.

Carcinoid Syndrome and Carcinoid Heart Disease

Two of our patients with colonic carcinoids and metastasis to the liver exhibited the carcinoid syndrome, and one of these also had carcinoid heart disease. None of our patients with metastasizing rectal carcinoids exhibited the syndrome, and there are no reported cases of rectal carcinoid with carcinoid syndrome in the literature.

Treatment and Results

In general, treatment consisted of either local excision of the lesion or radical resection of the rectum and colon together with adjacent involved tissues and corresponding lymphovascular bundle of the mesentery. Under the broad category of local excision, however, a variety of methods was used. Biopsy-forceps removal of the smallest lesions was considered adequate in many instances. It was possible, in some patients who had slightly larger tumors arising high in the rectum, to use cautery-snare removal for complete excision. For some lower lesions, less than 2 cm in diameter, and judged to be intramural in location, wide local surgical excision could be performed via either the transanal or transcoccygeal route.

Results in the surgical management of rectal carcinoids may be best described according to the size of the tumor. Of the 40 patients who had tumors less than 1 cm, all had local excisions. Thirty-two were living and well from 2 to more than 29 years; 3 less than 5 years; 8 from 5 to 10 years; 9 from 10 to 20 years; and 12 over 20 years. One in each of these categories died of a concurrent cancer of the cervix and rectum, and one died of coronary thrombosis, less than five years after removal of their rectal carcinoid. Five patients in this group were lost to follow-up. None died of their carcinoid.

Eight patients had lesions estimated to be greater than 1 cm and less than 2 cm in diameter. Six underwent local excision, and of these, four are living and well 6, 12, 15, and 25 years later. Another patient, a 36-year-old black woman, had a rectal carcinoid 1 cm in diameter with an adjacent satellite nodule 0.5 cm in size. Because of the radiographic documentation of a second tumor in the cecum, a laparotomy was performed and an anterior resection of the rectum done when it was discovered that the rectal tumor had metastasized to the mesenteric lymph nodes. A right hemicolectomy was also performed for what proved to be a large granular-cell myeloblastoma of the cecum. This patient is alive and well 18½ years after the operation. The remainder of this group (two patients) were lost to follow-up, but were free of disease when last heard from.

Fourteen patients whose rectal tumors were larger than 2 cm did poorly despite radical surgery. None lived more than five years after surgery; indeed 10 died of their disease less than one year from the time of treatment. The first manifestation of disease in five of these patients was a large liver metastasis; already these patients could not be helped by surgery, therapy, or chemotherapy. One patient had no specific record as to his original tumor size because his initial resection was done at another hospital. He succumbed to recurrent disease more than 10 years following original treatment.

The 12 patients with colonic carcinoids in general did poorly, and all but one had large tumors at the time of detection and treatment. The smallest tumor in this group measured 1½ cm and arose in the ileocecal region. Despite an ileocolectomy, the patient suffered from an unresectable liver metastasis 13 years after the original operation. The remaining 11 patients all had large tumors with serosal involvement; 4 of the 11 patients survived more than five years following resection. Two were alive and well when last heard from, and two others died of other causes without evidence of disease. Seven died of their disease under five years. The overall five-year survival for the patients with colonic carcinoids is thus 5/12 or 42%.

Based on this report and our study of carcinoids occurring in other anatomic sites from this institution (37,40,42), there is a definite correlation between pathologic and clinical presentation and expected result. Early tumors that are still located intramurally and are usually less than 2 cm (as can be detected by proctosigmoidoscopy) are usually asymptomatic and can be treated by adequate local excision, with excellent results. Conversely, more advanced carcinoid tumors, which have invaded the outer muscular wall or serosa and/or beyond, are usually more than 2 cm, are symptomatic, and are not often treated successfully, despite major surgical resection, radiotherapy, and treatment with various chemotherapeutic agents. Proctosigmoidoscopy and, more recently, colonoscopy, are two techniques that can detect the small and asymptomatic carcinoids. The removal of such early lesions can result in better control of this rare tumor.

ACUTE ANORECTAL COMPLICATIONS IN LEUKEMIC PATIENTS

A uniquely beneficial service can be rendered by the surgeon to leukemic patients with active disease who are suffering from acute anorectal complications, such as thrombosed and/or prolapsed, inflamed, ulcerated hemorrhoids, anal fissures, anal and perianal abscesses, anorectal fistulas, and so on, by resisting the normal impulse to operate on them. Indeed, strict avoidance of trauma to this sensitive anatomic area should be exercised by doctor and nurse alike in the avoidance of digital rectal examination, insertion of rectal thermometer, administration of enemas, and so on. These patients do not react normally to surgical intervention, as evidenced by the lack of wound healing, spreading sepsis, and increased bleeding due to alteration of their immunologic mechanisms and blood components (leukopenia, thrombocytopenia). Extensive necrosis of perianal and anorectal tissues, leading to death following incision and drainage, has been reported (43,46).

What has been efficacious for these patients in our experience (45) besides the usual supportive measures (analgesics, warm compresses, broad antibiotic therapy, etc.), is external irradiation (300 to 500 rads to the perineum in divided doses) via the cobalt machine. The same dose may be repeated in several days if the inflammatory condition persists. This modality of treatment can be particularly effective in the cellulitis stage. Abscesses that form may be drained through a minimal incision. Select conservative surgical therapy is used only in patients with chronic leukemia whose blood counts are near normal or normal, and in patients whose leukemia is in remission.

A current review (44) of adults with acute leukemia receiving massive myeloid depressant agents indicates an expectant remission response rate as high as 80% and the occurrence of acute anorectal complication as high as 20%. Conservative management as outlined above is recommended during the active phase of the blood disease, and elective surgery is advised during the remission phase, provided that the antileukemic drugs are stopped for several days before and after surgery.

REFERENCES

1. Goligher JC: Ca of the anal canal and anus, in *Surgery of the Anus, Rectum and Colon,* ed 3. Springfield, Ill: Charles C Thomas, pp 814–828.

2. Foraker AG, Miller CJ: Extramammary Paget's disease of perianal skin. *Cancer* 2:144, 1949.

3. Arminski TC, Pollard RJ: Paget's Disease of the anus secondary to a malignant papillary adenoma of the rectum. *Dis Colon Rectum* 16:46, 1973.

4. Williams SL, Rowgers LW, Quan SHQ: Perianal Paget's dis.: report of seven cases, *Dis Colon Rectum* 19:30–40, 1976.

5. Bowen JT: Precancerous dermatoses: A study of two cases of chronic atypical epithelial proliferation. *J Cut Dis* 30:241–255, 1912.

6. Quan SHQ, Pacheco L. Unpublished data, 1977.

7. Raaf JH, Krown SE, Pinsky CM, et al, Treatment of Bowen's disease with topical dinitrochlorobenzene and 5-fluorouracil. *Cancer* 37:1633–1642, 1976.

8. Scoma JA, Levy EI: Bowen's disease of the anus. *Dis Colon Rectum* 18:137–140, 1975.

9. Braastad FW, Dockerty MB, Dixon CF: Melano-epithelioma of the anus and rectum: Report of cases and review of literature. *Surgery* 25:82, 1949.

10. Husa A, et al: Anorectal malignant melanoma. A report of fourteen cases. *Acta Chir Scan* 140:66–72, 1974.

11. Pack GT, Oropeza R: A comparative study of melanoma and epidermoid ca of the A.C. a review of 20 m and 29 e.c. (1930–65). *Dis Colon Rectum* 10:161–176, 1967.

12. Quan SHQ, White JE, Deddish, MR: Malignant melanoma of the anorectum. *Dis Colon Rectum* 2:275–283, 1959.

13. Quan SHQ, Deddish MR: Noncutaneous melanoma: malignant melanoma of the anorectum. *Ca A Cancer Journal for Clinicians* 16:111–114, 1966.

14. Quan SHQ, Wanebo H. Unpublished data, 1978.

15. Sinclair DM, et al: Malignant melanoma of the anal canal. *Br J Surg* 57:808–811, 1970.

16. Smith LS Jr, Early detection and diagnosis of malignant melanoma pathology. Postgraduate course, #10. Comm on Cancer, Am College of Surgeons, 1977, pp 123–125.

17. Binkley GE: Epidermoid carcinoma of the anus and rectum. *Am J Surg* 79:90, 1950.

18. Morson BC, Pang, LSC: Anal cancer. *Proc Roy Soc Med* 61:623–625, 1968.

19. Newman HK, Quan SHQ: Multimodality therapy for epidermoid carcinoma of the anus. *Cancer* 37:12–19, 1976.

20. Nigro N, Vaitkevicius VK, Considine B: Combined therapy for cancer of the anal canal: a preliminary report. *Dis Colon Rectum* 17:354–356, 1974.

21. Quan SHQ, Magill GB, Leaming RH, Hajdu SI: Multidisciplinary preoperation approach to the management of epidermoid carcinoma of the anus and anorectum. *Dis Colon Rectum,* 21:89–91, 1978.

22. Stearns MW Jr: Epidermoid carcinoma of the anal region. *Am J Surg* 90:727, 1955.

23. Stearns MW Jr: Epidermoid carcinoma of the anal region. *Surg Gynec Obstet* 106:92, 1958.

24. Stearns MW Jr: Quan SHQ: Epidermoid carcinoma of the anorectum. *Surg Gynec Obstet* 131:953–957, 1970.

25. Wolfe HRI: The management of metastatic inguinal adenitis in epidermoid cancer of the anus. *Proc Roy Soc Med* 61:626–628, 1968.

26. Berg J, McNeer J: Leiomyosarcoma of the stomach: clinical and pathological study. *Cancer* 13:25, 1960.

27. Buckle AER, Evans L: Leiomyosarcoma of the rectum: report of a case. *Dis Colon :Rectum* 17:109, 1974.

28. Egeli R, Quan SHQ. Unpublished data, 1979.

29. Quan SHQ, Bader G, Berg JW: Carcinoid tumors of the rectum. *Dis Colon Rectum* 7:197–206, 1964.

30. Quan SHQ, Berg JW: Leiomyoma and leiomyosarcoma of the rectum. *Dis Colon Rectum* 5:415, 1962.

31. Warkel RL, Stewart JB, Temple AJ: Leiomyosarcoma of the colon: report of a case and analysis of the relationship of histology to prognosis. *Dis Colon Rectum* 18:501, 1975.

32. Bacon HE: *Cancer of the Colon, Rectum and Anal Canal.* Philadelphia, JB Lippincott Co, 1964, p 380.

33. Culp CE, Hill JR: Malignant lymphoma involving the rectum. *Dis Colon Rectum* 5:426–436, 1967.

34. Jackman RJ, Beahrs OH: Malignant lymphoma, in *Tumors of the Large Bowel.* Philadelphia, WB Saunders, 1968, pp 210–216.

35. Warren KW, Littlefield JB: Malignant lymphomas of the gastrointestinal tract. *Surg Clin* 35:735, 1955.

36. Wychulis AR, Beahrs OH, Woolner LB: Malignant lymphoma of the colon: a study of 69 cases. *Arch Surg (Chicago)* 93:215, 1966.

37. Hajdu SI, Winawer SJ, Myers WPL: Carcinoid tumors: A study of 204 cases. *Am J Clin Path* 61:1974.

38. Pearson CM, Fitzgerald PJ: Carcinoid tumors—reemphasis of their malignant nature; review of 140 cases. *Cancer* 2:1005, 1949.

39. Peskin GW, Orloff MJ: A clinical study of 25 patients with carcinoid tumors. *Surg Gynecol Obstet* 109:673, 1959.

40. Quan SHQ, Baker G, Berg JW: Carcinoid tumors of the rectum. *Dis Colon Rectum* 7:197–206, 1964.

41. Warren KW, Coyle EB: Carcinoid tumors of gastrointestinal tract. *Am J Surg* 82:372, 1951.

42. Zakariai YM, Quan SHQ, Hajdu SI: Carcinoid tumors of the gastrointestinal tract. *Cancer* 35:588–591, 1975.

43. Blank WA: Anorectal complications in leukemia. *Am J Surg* 90:738–741, 1955.

44. Hertz REL, Moffat R, Gee T. Unpublished data, 1978.

45. Sehdev, Mohan K, Dowling, MD Jr, et al: Perianal and anorectal complications in leukemia. *Cancer.* 31:149, 1973.

46. Walsh G, Stickley CS: Acute leukemia with primary symptoms in the rectum: A rapid increase in the white cells and fatal outcome. *South Med J* 96:684–689, 1934.

10

Radiation Therapy in the Clinical Management of Neoplasms of the Colon, Rectum, and Anus

Robert Leaming

In the management of neoplasms of the colon, rectum, and anus, surgical techniques have been extended as far as possible, so that with an average survival rate of 40 to 50%, adjuncts to surgery should be tried. Currently available adjuncts are radiation, chemotherapy, or immunotherapy, or combinations of these techniques.

Radiotherapy has not played a major role in the therapy for large-bowel cancer, except in rectal and anal cancer, which comprises about 40% of all colorectal cancer. The indications for radiotherapy are enumerated in Table 1.

CURATIVE THERAPY

If a patient refuses surgery or has a medical contraindication, radiotherapy may be administered as primary treatment. This may vary from intracavitary radiation to external radiotherapy, or some combination of the two. Intracavitary radiation as performed by Papillon (7) is limited to selected patients with polypoid, well-differentiated adenocarcinomas not exceeding 3 cm in diameter and located from 0 to 12 cm above the anal verge. This is contact therapy using 50 kV and for field sizes up to 3 cm in diameter. At this energy level penetration is limited and 1,500 to 2,000 rads are delivered for three to five applications in a period of four to six weeks. In a series of 133 patients treated by Papillon, 104 were free of disease with a five-year survival rate of 78%. Results in patients treated with electrofulguration reported by Madden and Kandalaft (4) and Crile and Turnbull (1) are given in Table 2. These are not strictly comparable because of the degree of selection in Papillon's series.

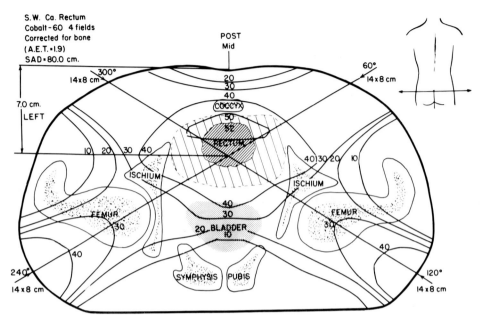

Figure 1. Isodose curves for curative radiotherapy for carcinoma of the rectum.

Curative radiotherapy by external sources requires careful treatment planning, which includes computerized tomographic (CT) scanning and simulation, from which the radiotherapist and physicist can accurately outline the area to be treated. This requires supervoltage units with accurate angulation and/or wedge application. Results with this method yield 5 to 10% five-year survival rates as reported by Williams and Horwitz (14) and Wang and Schultz (12). Figure 1 represents a treatment plan for curative radiotherapy as outlined above.

PALLIATION

The use of radiotherapy in a palliative effort has been described by numerous authors, but awareness of its beneficial effect is still lacking in many instances. Radiation is the most useful method of affording prompt, effective relief of pain from localized recurrence or inoperable cancer of the colon and anorectum. In any discussion of radiation of the G.I. tract we must consider tissue tolerance, including acute and late effects. Table 3 reveals the average tolerance by anatomical site.

At Memorial Hospital we have enthusiastically advocated the use of radiotherapy in a palliative sense. It has been used primarily for relief of pain and also to diminish bleeding and irritating discharge of inoperable rectal tumors and recurrent perianal malignant ulcerations. It has been employed regularly following unsuccessful attempts to resect primary or recurrent colorectal cancer, where residual tumor has been left behind. These areas are usually marked with metallic clips for portal localization. In 1965, a prospective study was started to evaluate our impressions (13). We have employed the concept of patterns and stages of disease as seen in Table 4.

Unless the patient has obvious abdominal carcinomatosis, we believe that most patients should be explored to determine nonresectability. If the neoplasms in such

Table 1. Indications for Radiotherapy

A. Curative—not indicated unless surgery is contraindicated
B. Palliation
   1. In unresectable primary lesions or recurrences
   2. For metastasis or malignant effusions
C. Adjuncts to surgery
   1. Preoperative
   2. Postoperative
   3. Intraoperative
   4. Combined treatment for anal epidermoid carcinoma

Table 2.

Author	Method	Number of Patients	Five-Year Survival Rate
Papillon (7)	Endocavitary contact therapy	133	78%
Crile and Turnbull (1)	Electrofulguration	62	68%
Madden (4)	Electrofulguration	110	58%

Table 3. Radiotherapy Tolerance by Anatomical Site

Small bowel	4,500 rads in 4–5 weeks
Colon	4,500 rads in 4–5 weeks
Rectum	6,000 rads in 6–7 weeks

Table 4. Concept of Patterns and Stages of Disease for the Large Bowel

	Stages		
Pattern	I Early Asymptomatic	II Progressive Compensated	III Progressive Decompensated
A. Localized	—	—	—
B. Hepatic	—	—	—
C. Intraabdominal	—	—	—
D. Generalized	—	—	—

Table 5. Radiotherapy for Local Disease
(103 Patients)

Response	Number	Percent
Excellent	27	26
Good	54	54
Fair	16	15
Poor	5	5

patients are found to be locally unresectable because of involvement of nerves, blood vessels, or other vital structures, and if an implant is not feasible, then the localized area of involvement is marked with clips for subsequent radiotherapy.

There were 103 patients with a local disease pattern, as seen in Table 5. These were patients with intrapelvic disease causing pain and pressure on the bladder, bowel, or sciatic nerve. A total of 80% of these patients experienced good or excellent response, and the average length of response after treatment in this group was 18 months. There were 22 patients, as seen in Table 6, with a hepatic pattern, where pain from progressive liver enlargement was a predominant symptom. Asymptomatic liver metastases were not treated by radiotherapy. Twelve of the 22 patients (50%) experienced good or excellent results with an average length of response. Obviously, there are too few patients in any subgroup to draw definite conclusions.

Patients with diffuse, gross, or miliary abdominal implants received radiotherapy at the site of bulky involvement that produced symptoms. In this group (Table 7) 16 of 27 patients (60%) received excellent or good palliation and the average length of response in this group was 11 months. Patients with a generalized pattern, that is, lung, brain, and bone metastases, received radiotherapy to localized areas for relief of symptoms. Liver metastases may also have been present but were not symptomatic. Six of 13 patients (Table 8) received a good or excellent response for an average of 8 months. In the estimation of response we used the Karnofsky method, based on the patient's objective and subjective response as well as performance status.

Dosage in these studies was modest; that is, 2,000 to 2,500 rads delivered in two to three weeks, except in liver metastases, where the usual dose was 3,500 rads in three to four weeks. Modest dosages of this magnitude may be repeated (except for liver metastases) to a total of three courses, which will afford further palliation over a substantial period of time with no significant side effects. Higher dosage has been considered, but in Table 9 comparison with other series using 4,000 to 6,000 rads indicates that the ultimate degree of significant palliation has been similar.

Table 6. Radiotherapy for Hepatic Disease
(22 Patients)

Response	Number	Percent
Excellent	2	9
Good	10	45
Fair	5	23
Poor	5	23

Table 7. Radiotherapy for Intraabdominal Disease (27 Patients)

Response	Number	Percent
Excellent	5	18
Good	11	41
Fair	7	26
Poor	4	15

Table 8. Radiotherapy for Generalized Disease (13 Patients)

Response	Number	Percent
Excellent	1	7
Good	5	40
Fair	4	30
Poor	3	23

Table 9. Comparison of Results of Local Palliation

	Institution or Author(s)				
	Memorial Hospital		Smedal et al. (10)		Wang and Schultz (12)	Williams et al. (15)
Response	Number	Percent	Number	Percent		
Excellent	27	26	13	26		
Good	54	54	12	24		
Fair	16	15	11	22		
Poor	5	5	14	28		
Machine used	Cobalt		2 MeV		Cobalt	1 MeV
Dose, rads	2,000		4,000–5,000		6,000	3,600–5,000
No. of patients	102		50		82	111
Significant palliation	80%		50%		87%	84%

Table 10. Survival and Dukes' Classification

Dukes' Classification	Number of Patients	Five-Year Survivors	Overall Five-Year Survival (%)
A			
Surgery	96	69	72
Radiation and surgery	103	75	73
B			
Surgery	145	92	63
Radiation and surgery	161	104	64
C			
Surgery	201	46	23
Radiation and surgery	195	72	37

ADJUNCT TO SURGERY

Preoperative

Radiation delivered before definitive surgery has been used at Memorial Hospital for many years. In 1961, we published the results of a retrospective review of the Memorial Hospital experience with preoperative irradiation in cancer of the rectum (3). This review recorded the findings in 1,876 patients with adenocarcinoma of the rectum and rectosigmoid from 1939 to 1951, as seen in Table 10. There was improvement in observed survival in Dukes' C patients from 23% with surgery alone up to 37% in those treated with preoperative irradiation. There was no significant effect in those without regional metastases. This study was not randomized, but there was a similar number of patients in each group, as demonstrated in Table 10.

On the basis of these studies, we renewed the use of preoperative irradiation in 1957, and in 1960 we began a randomized study, based on birthdate, which was terminated at the end of 1967 (11). All primary patients in whom curative resections were performed by members of the Rectal and Colon Service were included. The rectum and rectosigmoid were arbitrarily defined as the distal 16 cm of bowel measured by preoperative sigmoidoscopy. These patients received 2,000 rads in 10 treatments through

Table 11. Preoperative Irradiation in Rectal Carcinoma

	1939–1951	1957–1967
Total resected	971	790
No. of five-year survivors	479	468
Operative mortality		
Surgery alone	2.3%	2.4%
Irradiation and surgery	2.2%	5.3%
Survival with positive nodes		
Surgery alone	23%	45%
Irradiation and surgery	37%	45%

Table 12. Determinate Five-Year Survival

	1939–1951	*1957–1967*
Number of patients		
Surgery alone	473	414
Irradiation and surgery	498	376
Determinant five-year survival		
Surgery alone	47%	65%
Irradiation and Surgery	51%	67%

anterior and posterior pelvic portals measuring about 18 × 16 cm. Cobalt was used and surgery was performed from one day to six weeks after preoperative irradiation.

Table 11 compares the results of both series. Table 12 compares the determinant five-year survival with an without preoperative irradiation in the two series. The incidence of nodal involvement in the two series is compared in Table 13. Table 13 indicates that the incidence of nodal metastases was essentially the same whether or not preoperative irradiation had been given. This is important in view of the Veterans Administration (9) and the Yale (2) experiences, where a lower incidence of lymph-node metastases was found in those treated with radiation preoperatively, as seen in Table 14. These two studies indicate the value of preoperative irradiation, but only the V.A. study has enough patients to be statistically valid.

Survival rates of both sexes are compared in Table 15. The survival rate without preoperative irradiation was considerably higher in women than in men. This is a reflection of a generally better prognosis for women than for men. However, the survival of men and women who had preoperative irradiation was essentially the same. This might partially explain our differences from the V.A. study, since the patients in the V.A. study were exclusively males.

Site of failure, that is, local versus distant metastases, was studied as demonstrated in Table 16. In those without regional metastases there was no difference in the site of failure in the control or treated patients. However, when regional metastases were present there was a decrease in the percent due to local recurrence with a corresponding increase in failure due to distant metastases in those who were given preoperative irradiation. Because of the results of the second randomized study with preoperative irradiation, we no longer routinely deliver radiation prior to surgery. Its use is reserved for selected patients with clinically inoperable or borderline operable lesions.

Table 13. Incidence of Nodal Metastases

	1939–1951	*1957–1967*
Surgery alone	46%	37%
Irradiation and surgery	43%	35%

Table 14. Incidence of Nodal Metastasis in Other Series

Source	Surgery Alone	Irradiation and Surgery
V.A.	38%	24%
Yale	43%	22%

Postoperative

We and other groups are now interested in the evaluation of postoperative radiotherapy, particularly in the high-risk group. In these instances subclinical disease left at the time of surgery may be effectively controlled by early postoperative treatment. The use of postoperative radiotherapy has the following potential advantages:

1. Elimination of subclinical disease to prevent failures, which usually occur locally (50%) and early (within 7 months).
2. More accurate determination of the stage of disease would result in more meaningful assessment of objective therapy. Patients with favorable lesions as well as patient with liver metastases would not receive radiotherapy.
3. Use of metallic clips to delineate gross residual disease or suspicious margins.

Postoperative radiotherapy should be given as soon as the wound is healed, that is, from two to six weeks. The method of closure is important in that with primary closure, radiotherapy may begin after a minimum of two weeks, but with wounds that are packed open the delay may be as long as eight weeks. We are currently involved in two national studies that are considering adjuvant therapy, as seen in Table 17.

Intraoperative

Interstitial implants have been used occasionally, usually at the time of the reexploration for recurrent colorectal lesions when there is evidence of local disease which is nonresectable. Iodine[125] is at present used for permanent implants and irridum[192] for temporary implants. Size and proximity to vessels and other vital structures limit the indications for this modality.

Table 15. Survival Rates of Both Sexes, With and Without Preoperative Irradiation

	Surgery Alone		Irradiation and Surgery	
	Male	Female	Male	Female
Total number	218	196	225	151
Five-year survivors	114	128	126	87
% five-year survival	52%	65%	56%	57%

Table 16. Site of Failure and Preoperative Irradiation

	Negative Nodes		Positive Nodes	
	Surg. Alone	Surg. Plus Irrad.	Surg. Alone	Surg. Plus Irrad.
Total patients	172	180	79	107
Failures				
Local				
No.	18	14	24	17
%	10%	7.8%	30%	16%
Liver				
No.	7	10	9	11
%	4%	5.5%	11%	10%
Other[a]				
No.	10	12	11	31
%	6%	6.7%	14%	29%

[a] Other: lung, intraperitoneal, bone.

Combined Treatment for Anal Epidermoid Carcinoma

The results of radiotherapy or surgery alone in the management of anal carcinoma has been disappointing. These lesions often are highly anaplastic and are epidermoid carcinomas (or variants of epidermoid carcinoma), which are more radiosensitive than adenocarcinomas. In an attempt to improve our results we now use a multidisciplinary approach. These patients receive 5-FU daily for five days in the form of a continuous 24-hour infusion. Mitomycin C is given as a bolus injection on the first day. These patients then receive 3,000 rads in three weeks to the pelvis using cobalt therapy. This is followed by a surgical resection in 4 to 6 weeks. Table 18 represents a preliminary review of 18 patients with proven anal carcinoma and shows impressive responses after combined preoperative chemotherapy and radiotherapy.

Table 17. Two National Studies Considering Adjuvant Therapy

A. GI-6175: to compare survival and recurrence-free intervals following curative colonic resection for stages B$_2$ and C, radomized as follows:
  1. Control
  2. C. T.   MeCCNU plus 5-FU
  3. I. T.   MER
  4. I. T. + C. T.   Using above agents
B. GI-7175: to compare survival and recurrence-free intervals following curative resection for rectal carcinoma, stages B$_2$ and C, radomized as follows:
  1. Control
  2. R. T. alone   4,000–4,800 rads
  3. C. T. alone   5-FU + MeCCNU
  4. R. T. + C. T.   Using dose and agents above

Table 18. Tumor Reduction in Anal Carcinoma

Gross 50%	17/18
Microscopic carcinoma	7/18
No microscopic carcinoma	10/18

SUMMARY

The role of radiation therapy in the management of colorectal carcinoma is primarily adjunctive. Radiotherapy for definitive treatment can be expected to yield 5 to 10% five-year survivals. Its use as a palliative agent, especially in the relief of pain, produces favorable results in 50 to 80% and in our experience it is the most useful single agent in this regard. Radiotherapy as an adjunct still has advocates for preoperative use, but its value as a routine adjunct has not been shown by our experience. We are trying to assess the advantages of postoperative radiotherapy, where greater selection may be used.

We need to evaluate the efficacy of all modalities, including preoperative radiotherapy, for inoperable or borderline lesions, and postoperative radiotherapy to prevent local recurrence in high-risk groups plus chemotherapy and/or immunotherapy to aid in the control of distant metastases. Hopefully, national studies now under way will uncover the optimum modalities and sequence.

REFERENCES

1. Crile G Jr, Turnbull RB Jr: The role of electro coagulation in the treatment of carcinoma of the rectum. *Surg Gynecol Obstet* 135:391–396, 1972.
2. Kligerman MM, Urdaneta N, Knowlton A, et al: Preoperative irradiation of the rectosigmoid carcinoma, including its regional lymph nodes. *Am J Roentgenol Radium Ther Nucl Med* 114:498–503, 1972.
3. Leaming RH, Stearns MW Jr, Deddish MR: Preoperative irradiation in rectal carcinoma. *Radiology* 77:257–263, 1961.
4. Madden JL, Kandalaft S: Electro coagulation in the treatment of cancer of the rectum. *Surgical Annual* 6:195–212, 1974.
5. Nigro ND, Vaitkevicius VK, Considine B: Combined therapy for cancer of the anal canal: a preliminary report. *Dis Colon Rectum* 17:351–356, 1974.
6. Newman HK, Quan, SHQ: Multimodality therapy for epidermoid carcinoma of the anus. *Cancer* 37:12, 1976.
7. Papillon J: Intracavitary irradiation in early rectal cancer for cure: a series of 186 cases. *Cancer* 36(2):696–701, 1975.
8. Quan SHQ, Magill GB, Leaming RH, Hajdu S: Multidisciplinary preoperative approach to the management of epidermoid carcinoma of the anus and anorectum. *Dis Colon Rectum* 21(2):89–91, 1978.
9. Roswit B, Higgins GA, Humphrey EW, et al: Preoperative irradiation of operable adenocarcinoma of the rectum and rectosigmoid. *Radiology* 79:1, 1962.
10. Smedal MT, Wright KA, Siber FJ: The palliative treatment of recurrent carcinoma of the rectum and rectosigmoid with 2 MEV radiation: some results and description of a technique. *Am J Roentgenol* 100:904–908, 1967.
11. Stearns MW, Deddish MR, Quan SHQ, and Leaming RH. *Surg Gynecol Obstet* 138:584–586, 1974.

12. Wang CC, Schultz MD: The role of radiation therapy in the management of carcinoma of the sigmoid, rectosigmoid, and rectum. *Radiology* 79:1, 1962.

13. Whiteley HWJ, Stearns MW Jr, Leaming RH, Deddish MR: Palliative radiation therapy in patients with cancer of the colon and rectum. *Cancer* 25:343, 1970.

14. Williams IG, Horwitz H: The primary treatment of adenocarcinoma of the rectum by high voltage roentgen rays. *Am J Roentgenol* 76:9, 1956.

15. Williams IG, Schuleman IM, Todd IP: The treatment of recurrent carcinoma of the rectum by supervoltage x-ray therapy, *Br J Surg* 44:506, 1956.

11
A Chemotherapeutic Approach to Colorectal Carcinoma

Nancy Kemeny
Robert Golbey

INTRODUCTION

Large-bowel cancer afflicts more patients in the United States than any other malignant neoplasm, excluding skin cancer, and accounts for 15% of all cancer deaths (1). There has been little change in the past 30 years in the overall five-year survival rate, 45%, for patients who undergo curative surgical resection (2). At the time of initial surgery, almost half of the patients with colorectal carcinoma have some evidence of lymph-node involvement (3), and 10 to 25% of these patients already have liver metastases (4,5). To improve survival, effective treatment beyond surgical resection of the primary must be developed. This chapter will attempt to describe the role of chemotherapy in the management of large-bowel cancer.

5-Fluorouracil (5-FU) has been the drug of choice for the treatment of colorectal carcinoma for the last 20 years; the optimal dosage and route of administration are still controversial. Clinical trials using 5-FU alone, other single agents, and multiple-drug combinations will be reviewed. Special problems in the management of local, hepatic, and pulmonary metastases will be discussed and clinical trials of adjuvant chemotherapy in large-bowel cancer will be evaluated.

5-FLUOROURACIL

The first specific advance in the chemotherapy of large-bowel cancer was made by Heidelberger and coworkers (6), who developed 5-fluorouracil (5-FU) by substituting fluorine for the hydrogen in the 5 position of the uracil molecule. Some tumors incorporate uracil to a greater degree than normal tissues. The clinical usefulness of this agent was first reported by Ansfield (7), who obtained a 15% response rate with 5-FU in patients with colorectal carcinoma, using 15 mg/kg intravenously for five consecutive days and then half doses until toxicity (the standard loading dose). Twenty-three percent of the patients treated by this method suffered from severe leukopenia (W.B.C. < 2000 cells/mm^3) and 3% died from drug toxicity. A less toxic schedule was developed using 12 mg/kg intravenously for five consecutive days and is also referred to as the standard loading dose. Response rates were similar to the higher dose, but toxicity was much more manageable (8). Early work with the standard loading dose, mostly in very advanced disease, showed a great variation in response rate, 8–85% (8).

Oral Administration

Oral 5-FU was first used because it was more convenient for the patient. There was also evidence that oral 5-FU would possibly be more effective in treating hepatic metastases since it was delivered directly to the liver via the portal circulation (9,10). Douglass and Mittleman (11) demonstrated increased concentrations of 5-FU in the portal system after oral administration. Unfortunately, 5-FU has erratic and unpredictable gastrointestinal absorption (11,12). A randomized double-blind study (13) comparing oral with intravenous administration of 5-FU revealed a 12% and 26% response rate, respectively. Hepatic metastases also had a lower response with the oral method, 17%, versus 32% with the intravenous method. The average duration of response was 11 weeks for the oral method and 20 weeks for the intravenous method. Therefore, it appears that the oral administration of 5-FU is inferior, yielding fewer remissions of shorter duration.

Weekly Intravenous Administration

In an attempt to decrease toxicity and frequency of outpatient visits, 5-FU was administered weekly. The Western Cooperative Cancer Chemotherapy Group (14) used 15 to 20 mg/kg of 5-FU weekly and obtained a 28% total response rate. The Eastern Cooperative Oncology Group (15) used different schedules of weekly intravenous 5-FU, namely, 7.5, 15, and 20 mg/kg, and obtained objective responses in 6%, 20%, and 25% of the patients, respectively. Since hematologic toxicity was significantly more severe at the 20 mg/kg dose, the authors concluded that the optimal dose was 15 mg/kg. In order to evaluate the efficacy of various 5-FU schedules, the Central Oncology Group (16) randomized 270 patients to receive (1) 5-FU at 12 mg/kg administered for five consecutive days, followed by 11 half doses on alternate days until toxicity (standard loading dose), (2) a weekly intravenous dose of 15 mg/kg, (3) a weekly oral dose of 15 mg/kg, and (4) a "standard" low dose, 500 mg for four consecutive days and weekly thereafter. The response rates were 33%, 13%, 13%, and 14%, respectively. These data suggest that the weekly and oral methods of administration of 5-FU are inferior to the standard loading dose.

Continuous Intravenous Infusion

5-FU given by continuous 24-hour infusion produces significantly less hematologic toxicity than bolus injections of 5-FU (17). Hartman et al. (18) obtained a 23% response rate with the five-day continuous infusion. As a second treatment, after failure with weekly 5-FU, they obtained a 13% response rate. Seifert (19) randomized 70 patients with colorectal carcinoma to receive 5-FU by 24-hour continuous infusion versus the bolus administration, and obtained a 44% versus 22% response rate, respectively. It is important to note that patients were not stratified for sites of metastases; 55% of the bolus group had lung metastases, while these metastases were only present in 32% of the patients in the infusion group. Moertel and Reitemeier (8) had previously demonstrated the relationship between the site of metastases and response rate of 5-FU. In their results, lung metastases only responded at a rate of 6.4%, while 32% of the abdominal metastases and 24% of the liver metastases responded. Although the universality of this observation can be disputed, it does raise some question about the superiority claimed for the continuous 24-hour infusion method.

Summary

The average response rate for 5-FU in colorectal carcinoma is 21% (20) and the average duration of response is six months. Although the response rate and duration of response are low, the responders have a significant increase in survival (8). At high doses, 5-FU may have considerable toxicity, especially for patients with compromised hematopoietic reserve (7). The optimal dose to be used depends partially on the schedule of administration. A dose of 15 mg/kg seems to be the best for weekly administration, whereas 12 mg/kg is more appropriate for the standard loading dose method.

The oral method is clearly inferior to intravenous administration. Intravenous administration of 5-FU is probably best given by the standard loading dose. The 24-hour intravenous infusion method requires hospitalization, and the added expense may not be justified until it is clear that continuous infusion produces a higher response rate than the standard loading dose method. It is doubtful that any further manipulation of dose, schedule, or route of administration of 5-FU alone will produce any major therapeutic advance in colorectal carcinoma.

OTHER SINGLE AGENTS

No other single agent has produced a higher response rate than 5-FU. Of the agents tested, one of the more promising groups of drugs is the nitrosoureas: BCNU (1,3-bis(2-chloroethyl)-1-nitrosourea), CCNU (1-(2-chloroethyl)-3-cyclohexyl-1-nitrosourea), and MeCCNU (1-(2-chloroethyl)-3-4-methylcyclohexyl-1-nitrosourea). BCNU in a single or divided dose of 250 to 375 mg/m^2 produced a 13% (17/128) response rate, and up to 18% in patients with no prior chemotherapy. CCNU, at a lower dose of 130 mg/m^2 orally, achieved only a 9% response rate. MeCCNU, at a dose of 175 to 200 mg/m^2 orally, yielded an 11% (18/168) response rate, and up to 25% in previously untreated patients (21). A randomized trial at the Mayo Clinic (22) of 5-FU versus MeCCNU yielded a 14% and 25% response rate, respectively. MeCCNU is the preferred nitrosourea because of the convenience of oral administration, the higher response rate, and the longer duration of response: 5.5 months, compared to 4.5 months with CCNU and 2 months with BCNU (22).

Mitomycin C, an antibiotic developed from a culture of *Streptomyces caespitosus,* was introduced into clinical trials in Japan. Initial trials with the drug reported significant tumor regressions, but at the dose schedules used, severe toxicity was encountered (23). Subsequent modifications resulted in an acceptable level of toxicity. Three trials in the United States by Moertel et al. (24), Hum et al. (25), and Moore et al. (26) obtained 12%, 17%, and 24% response rates, respectively. In Hum's study, the mitomycin C was administered at 0.25 mg/kg weekly, and 43% of the patients developed thrombocyto-penia below 100,000 cells/mm^3. Although the overall response rate in colorectal carci-noma is 18% (27), the average duration of response appears to be only three to four months, and the margin between therapeutic dose and toxicity is narrow.

Many other chemotherapeutic agents have been evaluated, but none has shown consistently useful activity against colorectal carcinoma. Methotrexate has a reported response rate varying between 8% (28) and 41% (29). In a randomized study comparing intravenous methotrexate with 5-FU, there was a 10% and 29% response rate, respec-tively (30). Cis-diamminedichloroplatinum (cis-platinum) has been shown to have activity in many solid tumors, but so far has been ineffective in colorectal carcinoma. In a randomized study comparing cis-platinum, at a dose of 50 mg/m^2, with 5-FU, there was a 3% and 17.5% response rate, respectively (31). Using high-dose cis-platinum in previously treated patients, there were no responses in 19 patients (32). Adriamycin, which has produced significant responses in hepatoma and carcinoma of the stomach and gallbladder, has only a 9% response rate in colorectal carcinoma (33). In a ran-domized study of adriamycin versus 5-FU, the response rate was 13% and 24%, respec-tively (34). Cyclophosphamide has an average response rate of 21% in colorectal carcinoma (35), but the responses are usually very transient (36). DTIC (5-(3-dimethyl-1-triazeno)imidazole-4-carboxamide) at a dose of 4.5 mg/kg daily for 10 days produced a 13% (5/42) response rate (37).

Of the phase-II agents recently tested at Memorial Sloan-Kettering Cancer Center (MSKCC) on previously treated patients with colorectal carcinoma, 2,2'-anhydro-1-B-D-arabinofuranosyl-5-fluorocytosine (AAFC) (38) and Pyrazofurin (39), demonstrated no activity in this disease. Baker's antifol (40) and anguidine (41) both show minimal activity in previously treated patients with colorectal carcinoma, with response rates of about 10%.

COMBINATION CHEMOTHERAPY

The presently available chemotherapeutic agents used alone do not produce response rates above 25% or greatly prolong survival in patients with colorectal carcinoma. Com-bination chemotherapy has induced higher remission rates in leukemia, lymphomas, testicular and breast carcinoma and has been tried recently in the treatment of large-bowel cancer.

The Mayo Clinic (42) conducted a seven-arm stratified randomized trial in 132 patients with three active drugs, 5-FU, mitomycin C, and BCNU, to compare the effec-tiveness of these drugs when used alone or in double or triple combinations. 5-FU produced the highest response rate, 25%, while the other drugs alone or in combination yielded only a 5 to 18% response rate. In another study with mitomycin C and 5-FU administered by continuous infusion, the response rate for patients with metastatic colorectal carcinoma was 18% (43). The addition of cytosine arabinoside to mitomycin C and 5-FU did not increase the response rate (44).

Moertel et al. (45) combined MeCCNU, 170 mg/m^2 orally every 10 weeks, 5-FU, 10 mg/kg intravenously for 5 consecutive days and vincristine, 1 mg/m^2 intravenously on day one every 5 weeks (MOF). In a stratified, randomized study of this combination versus 5-FU alone, they obtained a 43% response rate with MOF and a 19% response rate with 5-FU. With a reduced dose of MeCCNU, 100 mg/m^2 monthly, Falkson and

Falkson (46) compared MOF with 5-FU in a randomized study and obtained a 33% response rate with MOF versus a 22% response rate with 5-FU. The Southwest Oncology Group (47) compared MeCCNU, 175 mg/m^2 every six weeks, plus 5-FU, 400 mg/m^2 I.V. weekly, versus the same dose and schedule of 5-FU alone in a randomized trial. Thirty-two percent of 152 patients responded with the combination, while only 10% responded with 5-FU alone. Two nonrandomized trials (48,49) using MeCCNU and 5-FU obtained response rates of 40% and 37%.

At MSKCC, a lower response rate was obtained with the MOF regimen, which may reflect variations in the definition of a response, the patient population, and/or the sites of metastases. A partial response (PR) is a greater-than-50% reduction in the sum of the products of two perpendicular diameters of all measurable lesions. The Mayo Clinic and the Southwest Oncology Group require only a 50% reduction in one measurable lesion and define a PR of malignant hepatomegaly as a 30% reduction in the sum of two measurements from the costal margin to the liver edge (45,47). In evaluating malignant hepatomegaly at MSKCC, the sum of measurements from the costal margin to the liver edge at 0, 5, 10, and 15 cm from the xiphoid is used and a 50% reduction in the sum is required to denote a PR. A minor response (MR) denotes a greater than 25% reduction in measurable disease. Abdominal and pelvic masses were rarely used as the only area of measurable disease at MSKCC (50) and represented about one-third of the indicator lesions in the studies from the Mayo Clinic, Falkson, and MacDonald (42,46,48). Abdominal metastases are associated with a higher response rate to chemotherapy, and their serial clinical measurement is subject to greater potential error than metastases to the lung (8,51).

At MSKCC, patients were randomized to one of two MOF regimens (A and B). The same total dose of MeCCNU, 150 mg/m^2, repeated every 10 weeks, was used as a single dose in MOF A or in equally divided doses for five consecutive days in MOF B. In both arms, 5-FU was administered at a dose of 300 mg/m^2 for five consecutive days every five weeks and vincristine at 1 mg/m^2 on day one of each cycle of 5-FU. The partial response rate was 10% in MOF A and 12% in MOF B. Minor response rates were 11% and 21%, respectively. Toxicity was greater in MOF A, with 40% of the patients experiencing vomiting and 30% severe thrombocytopenia, compared to only 3% and 7%, respectively with MOF B (50).

More recent studies using the MOF regimen have yielded response rates similar to those obtained at MSKCC. The Sidney Farber Cancer Center (52), using the same doses of MeCCNU and 5-FU used in the MSKCC study, obtained only two responses in 52 patients. A randomized study from Scotland (53), comparing MeCCNU and 5-FU with 5-FU alone, yielded a 16% versus 15% response rate, and a 22-versus 23-week median survival, respectively. The Southwest Oncology Group (43) combined MeCCNU with 5-FU by continuous infusion and obtained a 16% response rate. The Eastern Cooperative Oncology Group (ECOG) (54) randomized 640 patients with advanced colorectal carcinoma to receive (1) MeCCNU and 5-FU, (2) MOF, (3) MeCCNU, 5-FU, and dacarbazine, (4) MeCCNU, 5-FU, dacarbazine, and vincristine, and (5) 5-FU and hydroxurea. The response rates were 10%, 12%, 14%, 15%, and 21%, respectively. The median survival in weeks was 26, 33, 41, 40, and 33, respectively. This large study also confirms a lower response rate with the MOF regimen and shows no significant decrease in efficacy when vincristine was deleted from the combination. Moertel (55) recently reported on his expanded experience with the MOF combination and discovered a reduction of the initial response rates from 43% to 27%. In contrast to

Table 1. MeCCNU Plus 5-FU in Treatment of Colorectal Carcinoma

Investigators	MeCCNU mg/m²	5-FU mg	Vincr. mg/m²	Number of Patients	Partial Response, %
MacDonald (48)	150	500/m²	1	25	40
Posey (49)	175	12/m²	—	35	37
Falkson (46)	100	12/kg	1	46	37
Baker (47)	175	400/m²	—	152	32
Moertel (55)	175	10/kg	1	127	27
Buroker (43)	150	1000/m² over 24 h	—	133	16
Engstrom (54)	150	325/m²	1	81	12
Kemeny (50)	150	300/m²	1	69	11
Lokich (52)	150	300/m²	—	52	4
				Total: 679	Mean: 23.5%

the study from ECOG, Moertel observed a lower response rate, 16%, when vincristine was omitted.

Although early reports suggested that the MOF combination might be a significant advance in the treatment of metastatic colorectal carcinoma, recent studies have not confirmed these early high response rates. The mean response rate for 690 patients included in major clinical trials of the MOF regimen is 23.5% (Table 1). This overall response rate approximates that seen with 5-FU alone. However, in each of the three large randomized studies cited above (45,46,47), comparing MOF with 5-FU alone, there was a statistically significant increase in response rate with the MOF combination.

At MSKCC, the next chemotherapeutic trial in colorectal carcinoma was the addition of Streptozotocin to the MOF B combination (56). Streptozotocin, a nitrosourea with very little myelosuppressive effect, was administered at a dose of 500 mg/m² weekly. Of the 74 evaluable patients, 2 (3%) had a complete response (CR), 22 (29%) had a partial response (PR), and 13 (18%) had a minor response (MR). The PR and CR rates with the MOF-Streptozotocin was significantly higher than that obtained with the MOF combination, 32% and 11%, respectively ($p < 0.01$). The median survival of the partial responders, 14 months, was significantly higher than that of the nonresponders, 7 months ($p < 0.01$). If the entire patient population receiving MOF-Streptozotocin was compared to patients receiving the MOF combination, there was a significantly higher median survival, 11 versus 8 months, respectively ($p < 0.01$). However, responders in both the MOF and MOF-Streptozotocin studies had similar survival. The increase in survival with the MOF-Streptozotocin combination may represent an advance in the chemotherapeutic management of colorectal carcinoma. A prospective, randomized study comparing the two regimens is in progress at MSKCC.

SPECIAL PROBLEMS IN THE MANAGEMENT OF METASTATIC DISEASE

Local Disease

Fifty to seventy-five percent of patients who die of recurrent or metastatic colorectal cancer have local recurrence (57). Radical operative procedures have not prevented the local recurrence of cancer. The incidence of failure is directly related to the amount of bowel-wall penetration and/or lymph-node involvement (58,59). Gunderson and Sosin (60) tabulated the sites of recurrence in 74 patients with sigmoid or rectal carcinoma explored at varying intervals after initial curative surgery. The majority of recurrences were local; 38.8% of the patients had local metastases alone and 64.9% had local disease combined with distant metastases. The problem for the chemotherapist and the surgeon dealing with local recurrence is that it is usually not measurable or palpable. Physicians must then use the patient's symptoms as the chief indicator of local disease and improvement in these symptoms as the indicator of response.

Radiation therapy has been the treatment of choice in locally recurrent or unresectable colorectal carcinoma. In a study of 189 cases with pelvic disease, there was relief from the following symptoms following irradiation: pain in 77%, tenesmus in 73%, mucous discharge in 77%, and bleeding in 90% (61). In addition to palliative treatment, patients with clinically unresectable colorectal carcinoma may become operable following radiation. In a group of 44 patients considered inoperable, 27 were able to undergo complete resection after radiation, and 22 of these resected patients remained free of disease for a median followup of 27 months (62). The Mayo Clinic (63) compared radiotherapy and 5-FU treatment with radiotherapy and a placebo in patients with locally unresectable colorectal carcinoma. A total dose of 50 mg/kg of 5-FU was used at the onset of radiation. There was a median survival of 22.8 months for the patients receiving both treatments, versus 16.8 months for patients receiving radiation alone (p < 0.05). The mean duration of symptomatic control was also longer in the group receiving 5-FU and radiation.

At MSKCC, all patients with locally recurrent disease in the pelvis receive 3,000 rads to the pelvis over a three-week period and are then randomized to receive MeCCNU and 5-FU with or without Corynebacterium Parvum (C-Parvum), a nonspecific stimulator of the immune system. Twenty-six patients have been entered and their median survival currently is 12 months. It is too early to see whether C-Parvum is playing a role in extending survival. In summary, radiation therapy is useful in locally recurrent and pelvic disease both preoperatively to achieve resectability and for symptomatic palliation. The addition of 5-FU may increase the beneficial effect in this situation.

Hepatic Metastases

Liver metastases have been found in 10 to 25% of patients undergoing laparotomy for colorectal carcinoma (5) and in 59% of patients with advanced colorectal carcinoma (48). Patients with liver metastases from large-bowel cancer have an average survival of six months and without surgical intervention the five-year survival rate ranges from 1.5 to 8% (64,65). When assessing the prognosis and the results of treatment for liver metastases, it is important to relate survival to the extent of liver involvement with tumor. Patients with solitary metastases may have an average survival of 16 to 18 months without any treatment, while patients with wide-spread disease in both lobes have a survival of only three to five months (65,66).

In Foster's review (4) of the literature on 163 cases who underwent hepatic resection for liver metastases from colorectal carcinoma, 30% of the patients with solitary metastases survived for five years, while only 13% with multiple metastases survived for five years. At MSKCC (67), for patients with limited hepatic involvement who underwent liver resection, there was a 40% and 20% determinant 5- and 10-year survival rate, respectively. Most of the resected hepatic metastases were solitary, synchronous, and peripheral, allowing for treatment with simple wedge resection. Fortner et al. (68) reported a 72% three-year survival rate for 17 of 25 patients with hepatic resections for metastatic colorectal carcinoma. In the Mayo Clinic experience (69), there were no five-year survivors among patients with multiple metastatic lesions in the liver, but the 5- and 10-year survival rate after resection of solitary metastases was 42% and 28% respectively.

The indications for surgical resection of multiple liver metastases are not well defined. Because survival is so poor without treatment, one should consider systemic or intrahepatic infusion of chemotherapy. There have been no prospective randomized studies comparing the two methods. It has been reported that hepatic metastases derive 70–90% of their blood supply from the hepatic artery and little from the portal system (70). Although hepatic ligation has been noted to cause a reduction in the size of hepatic metastases and does frequently relieve the pain associated with rapidly progressive hepatomegaly, it has not produced a significant prolongation of survival (71). Hepatic artery infusion of antineoplastic drugs yields a 20–55% response rate with responders obtaining a median survival of 10–14 months compared to 4–8 months for nonresponders (72–75). There may be some benefit to infusing both the hepatic artery and portal vein (76), because it has been suggested that the portal vein nourishes the periphery of the tumor (77). Unfortunately, many of the studies employing hepatic artery infusion consider symptomatic improvement as a significant response, are uncontrolled, and deal with small numbers of patients. In some of these studies survival was calculated from the time of diagnosis and not from the initiation of treatment. At this time there is no direct evidence to suggest that hepatic infusion of chemotherapeutic agents is superior to systemic therapy. With the MOF-streptozotocin regimen used at MSKCC (56), 48% (27/56) of the patients with metastatic liver involvement responded to systemic chemotherapy. However, hepatic artery infusion may be of some value in patients whose hepatic tumor progresses while on systemic chemotherapy (73,77).

Surgical resection probably offers an increase in survival rates for patients with solitary liver metastases from colorectal carcinoma. It should be cautioned that studies claiming an increase in survival have been uncontrolled and have involved small numbers of patients. When the liver is involved with multiple metastatic nodules, it is generally accepted that surgical resection is not warranted. Intrahepatic infusion of chemotherapy or systemic chemotherapy are then the suggested therapeutic alternatives. Which method is superior is at present unresolved and is the subject of an ongoing prospective trial at MSKCC.

Pulmonary Metastases

The overall incidence of pulmonary metastases from colorectal carcinoma is about 14.5% (78). In a study of 185 patients followed up to 14 years after curative colorectal surgery, 3.2% developed solitary pulmonary nodules. Of these solitary nodules, four out of six were due to metastatic colorectal carcinoma and two were due to primary lung cancer (78). At MSKCC (79), in a group of 54 patients with colonic malignancy who developed synchronous or metachronous solitary lung nodules, only 25 proved to be metastatic colonic carcinoma, while the remaining cases represented either a new lung primary or benign disease. The reported five-year survival rate after surgical resection of solitary lung metastases from colorectal carcinoma is 28 to 35%, and 10-year survival rate is 16% with a median survival of 20 months (80). As in the case of solitary liver metastases, little has been written on the natural history of patients with solitary lung metastases who do not have pulmonary resections. Patients with generalized metastatic disease to multiple organs including the lung have a median survival of only 6 months. Therefore, at the present time it seems reasonable to resect solitary lung metastases, particularly if there is no other evidence of disease, since it is imperative to make a histologic diagnosis. A patient with multiple lung metastases should be given a trial of systemic chemotherapy. Our experience does not support Moertel's observation of a uniquely low response expectation for pulmonary metastases. In the MOF study, 31% of patients with pulmonary metastases responded, and in the MOF-Streptozotocin study, 40% responded (50,56).

ADJUVANT CHEMOTHERAPY

The use of chemotherapy in conjunction with primary curative surgery is conceptually appealing and has been successfully applied in Wilm's tumor, osteosarcoma, and choriocarcinoma. In mouse colon carcinomas, the addition of chemotherapy after surgical resection has increased survival (81). The initial human trials used intraoperative or immediate postoperative chemotherapy to sterilize cells liberated at surgery. One of the first studies compared thiotepa (into portal vein and intraperitoneally at surgery and intravenously postoperatively, employing a total dose of 0.8 mg/kg) with a placebo (82). There was no statistically significant difference in survival between the two groups, except for women over 55 years of age, in whom the seven-year survival rate was 65% for the treated group and 30% for the placebo group.

The Veterans Administration Surgical Adjuvant Group (VASAG) reported on three large randomized trials (83,84), one using 5-fluorodeoxyuridine (FUDR) and the other two using 5-FU (Table 1). In patients undergoing curative resection, there was no statistically significant increase in survival for the treated group. However, in all three studies the treatment arm had a slight advantage. The Eastern Cooperative Group (85) also found no increase in survival, although the disease-free interval was significantly longer ($p = .004$) for patients with a white blood cell count below 4,000 cells/mm^3, suggesting that chemotherapeutic toxicity may be necessary for the drug to be effective.

Rousselot (86), in a nonrandomized study, administered 5-FU directly into the isolated large bowel lumen at the time of surgery, followed by two additional doses of 5-FU intravenously, and reported a 58% eight-year survival in patients with Dukes' C lesions. On the other hand, Lawrence (87) in a randomized trial using the technique described by Rousselot, plus monthly courses or oral 5-FU, found no difference in survival between the treated and non-treated groups at five years, 58% versus 56% (Table 2).

Two nonrandomized trials using adjuvant chemotherapy in patients with Dukes' B and C colorectal carcinoma suggest that there is an increase in survival for the treated patients. Using two five-day courses of intravenous 5-FU, Li and Ross (88) reported a five-year survival of 82% and 58% for patients with Dukes' B and C lesions, respectively. He compared these results with those of historical control groups of patients in the same institution whose survival was 59% and 24%, respectively. Mavligit et al. (89) found no difference in the survival time between patients treated with Bacillus Calmette-Guerin (BCG) or BCG plus 5-FU. When they compared the treated groups with his-

Table 2. Colorectal Carcinoma Adjuvant Chemotherapy

| | | | Survival % at 5 yrs | |
| | | Evaluable | | |
Study	Drug	Patients	Treated	Control
VASAG (81)	Thiotepa 0.8 mg/kg total dose	177	57	45
		♀ > 55	65	30[a]
VASAG (82)	FUDR 20 mg/kg × 3 days, then at 6 weeks 30 mg/kg loading dose	735	50	47
VASAG (83)	5-FU 12 mg/kg × 5 days, repeated once in 6 weeks	308	59	49
VASAG (83)	5-FU 12 mg/kg × 5 days, then every 6–8 weeks for 1½ yr	522	49	44
Lawrence (87)	5-FU 30 mg/kg intraluminal, then loading dose 5-FU orally for 1 year	203	58	56
COG (84)	5-FU 12 mg/kg loading dose, then weekly 12 mg/kg for 1 yr	337	74	72[b]

[a] Survival: 7 yr.

[b] Survival: 2 yr.

torical control groups of untreated patients, they found that the survival of the Dukes' C chemotherapy group almost overlapped the curve of the Dukes' B historical control group. However, both studies were retrospective and the lack of concomitant controls prevents definitive conclusions.

The importance of randomized controls in adjuvant studies is demonstrated in a study by VASAG (84). In two separate randomized trials using 5-FU adjuvant chemotherapy for colorectal carcinoma, there was no statistical difference between the treated and untreated patients, but there was an increase in survival in the placebo group from 16% in 1971 to 27% in 1976. If the 1976 chemotherapy trial had used the 1971 historical control for comparison, the authors might have concluded that there was a significant improvement in survival with the use of 5-FU. This sequential study illustrates the hazard of using historical controls.

Table 2 lists the major prospective randomized studies of adjuvant chemotherapy for colorectal carcinoma. In none of these studies was there a significant increase in survival

Table 3. Gastrointestinal Tumor Group Protocols for Adjuvant Chemotherapy of Colorectal Carcinoma

After Curative Colon Resection, Randomized to:	After Curative Rectal Resection, Randomized to:
1. Control	1. Control
2. MeCCNU and 5-FU	2. Radiotherapy (4,000 rads)
3. MER[a]	3. MeCCNU and 5-FU
4. MeCCNU and 5-FU plus MER	4. Radiotherapy plus MeCCNU and 5-FU

[a] Methanol extraction residue of BCG.

for the treated group. However, in all the studies, the treated group fared slightly better than the control group. It is possible that a therapeutic advantage for chemotherapy was missed because the sample size was not large enough (90).

At MSKCC, patients with Dukes' C colorectal carcinoma are entered into one of the two Gastrointestinal Tumor Study Group protocols outlined in Table 3. It is too early to draw conclusions from these studies. To date, there is no evidence from prospective randomized studies that any adjuvant chemotherapy used so far in colorectal carcinoma has any major effect. Perhaps as more effective combinations for metastatic disease are developed, better results with adjuvant chemotherapy will be achieved.

REFERENCES

1. Silverberg E, Holleb AI: Cancer statistics. *Cancer* 21:13, 1971.

2. Silverberg E: Cancer Statistics. *Cancer* 27:26, 1977.

3. Coller FA: *Cancer of the Colon and Rectum.* New York, American Cancer Society, Inc., 1956.

4. Foster JH: Survival after liver resection for secondary tumors. *Am J Surg* 135:389, 1978.

5. Bengmark S, Hafstrom L: The natural history of primary and secondary malignant tumors of the liver. *Cancer* 23:198, 1969.

6. Heidelberger C, Chaudhuri NK, Danneberg P, et al: Fluorinated pyrimidines, a new class of tumour-inhibitory compounds. *Nature* 179:663, 1957.

7. Ansfield F, Schroeder JM, Curreri AR: Five years experience with 5-fluorouracil. *JAMA* 181:295, 1962.

8. Moertel CG, Reitemeier RJ: *Advanced Gastrointestinal Cancer-Clinical Management and Chemotherapy.* New York, Harper & Row, 1969.

9. Khung CL, Hall TC, Piro AJ, et al: A clinical trial of oral 5-fluorouracil. *Clin Pharmacol Ther* 7:527, 1966.

10. Lahiri SR, Bioleau G, Hall TC: Treatment of metastatic colorectal carcinoma with 5-fluorouracil by mouth. *Cancer* 28:902, 1971.

11. Douglass HO Jr, Mittleman A: Metabolic studies of 5-fluorouracil-II. Influence of the route of administration on the dynamics of distribution in man. *Cancer* 34:1878, 1974.

12. Cohen JL, Irwin LE, Marshall GJ, et al: Clinical pharmacology of oral and intravenous 5-fluorouracil (NSC-19893). *Cancer Chemother Rep* 58:723, 1974.

13. Hahn RG, Moertel CG, Schutt AJ, et al: A double-blind comparison of intensive course 5-fluorouracil by oral vs. intravenous route in the treatment of colorectal carcinoma. *Cancer* 35:1031, 1975.

14. Jacobs EM, Reeves WJ, Wood DA, et al: Treatment of cancer with weekly intravenous 5-fluorouracil. *Cancer* 27:1302, 1971.

15. Horton J, Olson KB, Sullivan J, et al: 5-fluorouracil in cancer: An improved regimen. *Ann Intern Med* 73:897, 1970.

16. Ansfield F, Klots J, Nealon T, et al: A phase III study comparing the clinical utility of four regimens of 5-fluorouracil. *Cancer* 39:34, 1977.

17. Clarkson RB, O'Connor A, Winston L, et al: The physiologic disposition of 5-fluorouracil and 5-fluoro-2'deoxyuridine in man. *Clin Pharmacol Ther* 5:581, 1964.

18. Hartman HA, Jr, Kessinger MA, Lemon HM, et al: Five-day continuous infusion of 5-FU for advanced colorectal adenocarcinoma. *Proc Am Assoc Clin Oncol* 19:368, 1978.

19. Seifert P, Baker LH, Reed MD, et al: Comparison of continuously infused 5-fluorouracil with bolus injection in treatment of patients with colorectal adenocarcinoma. *Cancer* 36:123, 1975.

20. Krakoff IH: Chemotherapy of gastrointestinal cancer. *Cancer* 30:1600, 1972.

21. Wasserman TH, Slavik M, Carter SK: Clinical comparison of the nitrosoureas. *Cancer* 36:1258, 1975.

22. Moertel CG: Therapy of advanced gastrointestinal cancer with the nitrosoureas. *Cancer Chemother Rep* (Part 3) 4:27, 1973.

23. Frank W, Osterberg AE: Mitomycin C (NSC-26980): An evaluation of the Japanese reports. *Cancer Chemother Rep* 9:114, 1960.

24. Moertel CG, Reitemeier RJ, Hahn RG: Mitomycin C therapy in advanced gastrointestinal cancer. *JAMA* 204:1045, 1968.

25. Hum GJ, Bogdon DL, Bateman JR: Phase I-II evaluation of weekly mitomycin C (NSC-26980) for patients with metastatic GI and breast malignancies. *Oncology* 30:236, 1974.

26. Moore GE, Bross IDJ, Ansman R, et al: Effects of mitomycin in 346 patients with advanced cancer. *Cancer Chemother Rep* 52:675, 1968.

27. Crooke ST, Bradner WT: Mitomycin C: A review. *Cancer Treat Rev* 3:121, 1976.

28. Moertel CG, Reitemeier RJ, Hahn RG: Oral methotrexate therapy of gastrointestinal carcinoma. *Surg Gynecol Obstet* 130:292, 1970.

29. Sullivan RD, Miller E, Zurek WZ, et al: Re-evaluation of methotrexate as an anticancer drug. *Surg Gynecol Obstet* 127:819, 1967.

30. Eastern Cooperative Group in Solid Tumor Chemotherapy: Comparison of antimetabolites in the treatment of breast and colon cancer. *JAMA* 200:770, 1967.

31. Kovach JS, Moertel CG, Schutt AJ, et al: Phase II study of cis-diamminedichloroplatinum (NSC-119875) in advanced carcinoma of the large bowel. *Cancer Chemother Rep* 57:357, 1973.

32. Samal B, Vainutis V, Singhakowinta A, et al: Cis-diamminedichloroplatinum (CDDP) in advanced breast and colorectal carcinomas. *Proc Am Assoc Clin Oncol* 19:347, 1978.

33. Carter SK, Friedman M: Integration of chemotherapy into combined modality treatment of solid tumors II. Large bowel carcinoma. *Cancer Treat Rep* 1:111, 1974.

34. Frytak S, Moertel CG, Schutt AJ, et al: Adriamycin (NSC-123127) therapy for advanced gastrointestinal cancers. *Cancer Chemother Rep* 59:405, 1975.

35. Carter SK: Cyclophosphamide in solid tumors. *Cancer Treat Rep* 2:295, 1975.

36. Schutt AJ, Hahn RG, Reitmeier RJ, et al: A phase II study of intermittent high-dose cyclophosphamide therapy of advanced gastrointestinal cancer. *Cancer Res* 33:2218, 1973.

37. Slavik M: Clinical studies with DTIC in various malignancies. *Cancer Treat Rep* 60:213, 1976.

38. Kemeny N, Yagoda A, Burchenal JH: Phase II study of 2,2′-anhydro-1-B-D-arabinofuranosyl-5-fluorocytosine (AAFC) in advanced colorectal carcinoma. *Cancer Treat Rep* 62:463, 1978.

39. Carroll D, Kemeny N, Gralla R: Phase II evaluation of pyrazofurin in patients with advanced colorectal carcinoma. *Cancer Treat Rep* 63:139, 1979.

40. Padilla F, Correa J, Buroker T, et al: Phase II study of Baker's antifol in advanced colorectal cancer. *Cancer Treat Rep* 62:553, 1978.

41. Murphy WK, Burgess MA, Valdivieso M, et al: Anguidine: An early phase II study in colorectal adenocarcinoma. *Proc Am Assoc Clin Oncol* 19:411, 1978.

42. Reitemeier RJ, Moertel CG, Hahn RG: Combination chemotherapy in gastrointestinal cancer. *Cancer Res* 30:1425, 1970.

43. Buroker T, Kim PN, Groppe C, et al: 5-FU infusion with Methyl-CCNU in the treatment of advanced colon cancer. *Cancer* 42:1228, 1978.

44. De Jager R, Magill GB, Golbey RB, et al: Mitomycin C, 5-fluorouracil and cytosine arabinoside (MFC) in gastrointestinal cancer. *Proc Am Soc Clin Oncol* 15:178, 1978.

45. Moertel CG, Schutt AJ, Hahn RG, et al: Therapy of advanced colorectal cancer with a combination of 5-fluorouracil, methyl-1-2 cis(2-chlorethyl)-1-nitrosourea, and vincristine, brief communication. *J Natl Cancer Inst* 54:69, 1975.

46. Falkson G, Falkson H: Fluorouracil, methyl-CCNU and vincristine in cancer of the colon. *Cancer* 38:1468, 1976.

47. Baker LH, Talley RW, Matier R, et al: Phase III comparison of the treatment of advanced gastrointestinal cancer with bolus weekly 5-FU vs. methyl CCNU plus bolus weekly 5-FU. *Cancer* 38:1, 1976.

48. MacDonald JS, Kisner DF, Smythe T, et al: 5-fluorouracil (5-FU), methyl CCNU and vincristine in the treatment of advanced colorectal cancer. Phase II study utilizing weekly 5-FU. *Cancer Treat Rep* 60:1597, 1976.

49. Posey LE, Morgan LR: Methyl CCNU versus Methyl CCNU and 5-fluorouracil in carcinoma of the large bowel. *Cancer Treat Rep* 61:1453, 1977.

50. Kemeny N, Yagoda A, Golbey RB: A randomized study of two different schedules of Methyl CCNU, 5-FU and vincristine for metastatic colorectal carcinoma. *Cancer*, 43:78, 1979.

51. Moertel CG, Hanley JA: The effect of measuring error on the results of therapeutic trials in advanced cancer. *Cancer* 38:388, 1976.

52. Lokich JJ, Skarin AT, Mayer RJ, et al: Lack of effectiveness of combined 5-fluorouracil and Methyl CCNU therapy in advanced colorectal cancer. *Cancer* 40:2796, 1977.

53. Abdallah AM, Soukop M, Bell G, et al: A controlled study of 5-fluorouracil versus 5-fluorouracil and Methyl CCNU in advanced gastrointestinal adenocarcinoma. *Clin Oncol* 3:247, 1977.

54. Engstrom P, MacIntyre J, Douglass H Jr, et al: Combination chemotherapy of advanced bowel cancer. *Proc Am Assoc Clin Oncol* 19:384, 1978.

55. Moertel C: Chemotherapy of gastrointestinal cancer. *N Engl J Med* 229:1049, 1978.

56. Kemeny N, Yagoda A, Golbey R: Methyl CCNU (MeCCNU), 5-fluorouracil (5-FU), vincristine and Streptozotocin (MOF-STREP) for metastatic colorectal carcinoma. *Proc Am Assoc Clin Oncol* 19:354, 1978.

57. Gunderson L: Combined irradiation and surgery for rectal and sigmoid carcinoma. *Curr Prob Cancer* 1:40, 1976.

58. Gabriel WB, Dukes C, Bussey HJR: Lymphatic spread in cancer of the rectum. *Br J Surg* 23:395, 1935.

59. Astler VB, Coller FA: The prognostic significance of direct extension of carcinoma of the colon and rectum. *Ann Surg* 139:846, 1954.

60. Gunderson LL, Sosin H: Areas of failure found at reoperation (second or symptomatic look) following "curative surgery" for adenocarcinoma of the rectum: Clinicopathologic correlation and implications for adjuvant therapy. *Cancer* 34:1278, 1974.

61. Williams IG, Horwitz H: The primary treatment of adenocarcinoma of the rectum by high voltage roentgen rays (1,000 kV). *Am J Roentgenol Radium Ther Nucl Med* 76:919, 1956.

62. Pilepich MV, Munzenrider JE, Tak WK, et al: Preoperative irradiation of primarily unresectable colorectal carcinoma. *Cancer* 42:1077, 1978.

63. Carter SK: Current protocol approaches in large bowel cancer. *Semin Oncol* 3(4):433, 1976.

64. Abrams MS, Lerner HJ: Survival of patients at Pennsylvania Hospital with hepatic metastases from carcinoma of the colon and rectum. *Dis Colon Rectum* 14:431, 1971.

65. Wood CB, Gillis CR, Blumgart LH: A retrospective study of the natural history of patients with liver metastases from colorectal cancer. *Clin Oncol* 2:285, 1976.

66. Neilsen J, Balsey J, Jensen HE: Carcinoma of the colon with liver metastasis. *Acta Chir Scand* 137:463, 1971.

67. Attiyeh FF, Wanebo HJ, Stearns MW Jr: Hepatic resection for metastasis from colorectal cancer. *Dis Colon Rectum* 21:160, 1978.

68. Fortner JG, Kim DK, Maclean BJ, et al: Major hepatic resection for neoplasia: Personal experience in 108 patients. *Ann Surg* 188:363, 1978.

69. Wilson SM, Adson MA: Surgical treatment of hepatic metastases from colorectal cancers. *Arch Surg* 111:330, 1976.

70. Breedis C, Young C: The blood supply of neoplasms in the liver. *Am J Pathol* 30:969, 1954.

71. Nilsson LA: Therapeutic hepatic artery ligation in patients with secondary liver tumors. *Rev Surg* 6:374, 1966.

72. Cady B, Oberfield RA: Regional infusion chemotherapy of hepatic metastases from carcinoma of the colon. *Am J Surg* 127:220, 1974.

73. Ansfield FJ, Guillermo R, Davis HI, et al: Further clinical studies with intrahepatic arterial infusion with 5-fluorouracil. *Cancer* 36:2443, 1975.

74. Watkins E Jr, Khazei AM, Nahra KS: Surgical basis for arterial infusion chemotherapy of disseminated carcinoma of the liver. *Surg Gynecol Obstet* 130:580, 1970.

75. Fortner JG: Current management of tumors of the liver. *Surg Clin North Am* 57:465, 1977.

76. Taylor I: Cytotoxic perfusion for colorectal liver metastases. *Br J Surg* 65:109, 1978.

77. Ramming KP, Sparks FC, Eilber FR, et al: Management of hepatic metastases. *Sem Oncol* 4:71, 1977.

78. Schulten MF, Heiskell CA, Shields TW: The incidence of solitary pulmonary metastasis from carcinoma of the large intestine. *Surg Gynecol Obstet* 143:727, 1976.

79. Cahan WG, Castro EB, Hajdu SI: The significance of a solitary lung shadow in patients with colon carcinoma. *Cancer* 33:414, 1974.

80. McCormack PM, Bains MS, Beattie EJ Jr, et al: Pulmonary resection in metastatic carcinoma. *Chest* 73:163, 1978.

81. Corbett TH, Griswold DP, Roberts DVM, et al: Evaluation of single agents and combinations of chemotherapeutic agents in mouse colon carcinomas. *Cancer* 40:2660, 1977.

82. Holden WD, Dixon WJ, Kuzma JW: The use of triethylenethiophosphoramide as an adjuvant to the surgical treatment of colorectal carcinoma. *Ann Surg* 165:481, 1967.

83. Dwight RW, Humphrey EW, Higgins GA, et al: FUDR as an adjuvant to surgery in cancer of the large bowel. *J Surg Oncol* 5:243, 1973.

84. Higgins GA, Humphrey E, Juler GL, et al: Adjuvant chemotherapy in the surgical treatment of large bowel cancer. *Cancer* 38:1461, 1976.

85. Grage TB, Metter GE, Cornell GN, et al: Adjuvant chemotherapy with 5-fluorouracil after surgical resection of colorectal carcinoma. *Am J Surg* 133:59, 1977.

86. Rousselot LM, Cole DR, Grossi CE, et al: Adjuvant chemotherapy with 5-fluorouracil in surgery for colorectal cancer: eight year report. *Dis Colon Rectum* 15:169, 1972.

87. Lawrence W Jr, Terz JJ, Horsley S III: Chemotherapy as an adjuvant to surgery for colorectal cancer. *Arch Surg* 113:164, 1978.

88. Li MC, Ross ST: Chemoprophylaxis for patients with colorectal cancer—prospective study with five-year follow-up. *JAMA* 235:2825, 1976.

89. Mavligit GM, Gutterman JU, Malahay MA: Adjuvant immunotherapy and chemoimmunotherapy in colorectal cancer (Dukes' class C). *Cancer* 40:2726, 1977.

90. Freiman JA, Chalmers TC, Smith H Jr, et al: The importance of beta, the type II error and sample size in the design and interpretation of the randomized control trial. *N Engl J Med* 299:690, 1978.

12

A Review of Immunologic Reactivity in Patients with Colorectal Cancer

Harold J. Wanebo

The immune response can be functionally divided into cell-mediated (delayed type) and humoral or antibody-mediated segments (1). The components of the cell-mediated system include thymus-dependent lymphocytes and macrophages (reticuloendothelial cells). The humoral immune system is composed of bone-marrow–derived lymphocytes (precursors to antibody-producing plasma cells) and the myriad of cells involved in production of complement (2). Animal experiments and observations of naturally occurring specific immune deficits in humans have defined the anatomic locations of thymus-dependent and bone-marrow–dependent lymphocytes and lymph nodes. Thymus-dependent lymphocytes are concentrated in the paracortex, where they respond to antigenic stimulation by proliferation (3,4); bone-marrow–dependent lymphocytes are found in germinal centers and their progeny plasma cells in the medullary cord (3,5–7). The proliferation of lymphocytes that occurs in both the paracortex and germinal centers of lymph nodes following grafting with tumors and allogeneic skin grafts, seems to correlate with cellular or humoral immune responses, respectively (3,8,9).

IMMUNOMORPHOLOGY

Black, Kerpe, and Speer, in 1953, first called attention to the favorable prognostic significance of a reactional pattern, termed *sinus histiocytosis,* in the regional lymph nodes of breast-cancer patients (10). According to Black and coworkers, the highest survival rate occurred in patients with maximum sinus histiocytosis, whereas poorer survival rates were recorded in those with lesser degrees of histiocytic activity in the sinusoids (10,11). Patt et al have recently conducted an immunomorphologic study of the mesenteric lymph nodes draining sigmoid colon cancer (12). They found that patients whose lymph nodes showed morphologic evidence of cell-mediated immunity, as manifested either by an increased number of paracortical immunoblasts or sinus histiocytosis, survived longer than those whose lymph nodes showed no such changes (12), and that patients whose lymph nodes showed simultaneous paracortical activity and sinus histiocytosis had the best survival. Not only did this favorable lymph-node histology appear to be independent of the extent of the primary tumor, as determined by Dukes' classification, but the five-year survival rate was also improved in patients with Dukes' B and C lesions who had sinus histiocytosis and/or abundant paracortical immunoblasts. Histologic parameters that suggested an antibody-mediated immune response, that is, germinal center activity, were not found to be an important prognostic indicator. These findings were at variance with those of Tsakraklides et al, who found no significant improvement in survival of patients whose mesenteric nodes showed signs of increased T-cell activity (lymphocyte predominance pattern), but did find marginal improvement in patients with prominent germinal center activity in the regional nodes (factors suggesting increased B-cell activity). Although the reasons for these differences are not clear, they may be related to sampling; that is, Patt et al limited their study to the sigmoid colon, whereas Tsakraklides et al studied the entire left colon and rectum (12,13).

Lymphocyte infiltration in tumor tissue was first recognized as having prognostic importance in gastric cancer by McCarty and Mahle in 1921 (14), and in breast cancer by Moore and Foote (15). Subsequently, Sion and Friedell (16) studied the morphology of 117 patients with colon cancer and 54 patients with colonic polyps and found that lymphocytic infiltration was easily demonstrated in the benign polyps, but was either absent or sparse in the invasive cancer. The deeper the invasion of the cancer, the sparser was the lymphocyte infiltrate. It is of interest that there were nine cases with polyps adjacent to the invasive cancer, whose abundant lymphocyte infiltrates contrasted with the absence of lymphocyte infiltrates in the cancer. These effects may in part be related to the depressive impact of the cancer on the tissue lymphocytes, as reported by Nind et al (17). Pihl et al semiquantitated perivascular lymphocyte cuffing in the tissue adjacent to the primary tumors and the paracortical hyperplasia in regional lymph nodes in patients with Dukes' B cancer. These two factors, where combined, correlated with favorable disease-free interval and survival rates (18).

GENERAL IMMUNE REACTIVITY IN PATIENTS WITH COLORECTAL CANCER*

Lymphocyte Levels and Subpopulations

Depressed lymphocyte counts in patients with neoplastic disease have been associated with a poor prognosis (19). Kim et al studied the association between the pretreatment lymphocyte count and five-year survival in patients with colorectal cancer (20). Some 188 patients with five-year followup showed a significant difference in the survival rate in relation to the lymphocyte count: 61% for patients with counts greater than 2,000 cells/mm^3 versus 30% for those with counts less than 1,000 cells/mm^3 and 58% for the intermediate group ($p < 0.05$). Patients with Dukes' B and C lesions and lymphocyte counts over 2,000 cells/mm^3 demonstrated a survival rate of 81%, compared with 50% for those with lower counts. Of note, women had significantly higher lymphocyte counts

* See Table 1.

Table 1. Tests of General Immune Competence

In Vivo—Delayed Hypersensitivity Tests

Primary tests (de novo sensitivity)
    DNCB   (2,4-dinitrochlorobenzene)
    KLH   (key hole limpet hemocyanin)

Recall tests
    Candida albicans
    Dermatophytin
    Streptokinase-Streptodornase (SK-SD)
    Mumps
    Tuberculins

In Vitro Tests

Cellular factors
    Total lymphocyte–monocyte levels
        T cells (Total rosette forming cells; active rosette forming cells)
        B cells (Surface IgG, receptors for Fc and complement)
Null cells (Non-T or B, includes K cells)
Monocytes (Stain with esterase, Fc and C_3 receptors)
    Lymphocyte function
        Blastogenesis
            Mitogens (PHA, PWM, Con A)
            Antigens (*S. aureus, C. albicans, E. coli,* SK-SD, tuberculin, mumps virus)
            Alloantigens (allogeneic lymphocytes)
        Lymphokine production (MIF)
            Cytotoxicity: direct, antibody dependent
    Monocyte–macrophage function
        Chemotaxis
        Cytotoxicity (tumor cell, ADCC)
        Phagocytosis
        Enzyme production, i.e., lysozyme
    Granulocyte function
        Nitroblue tetrazolium
        Bacterial phagocytosis—killing
Humoral factors
    Immunoglobulin levels—IgG, IgA, IgM
        Antibody response
            KLH—primary and secondary response
            S. typhi
            Influenza
        Complement
            Total
            Components, i.e., C_1q, C_3
            Complexes (Raji method, C_1q method)

---

and higher survival rates than men, both as a group and within each stage (20). Kim et al. noted that although the lymphocyte count varied between stages, there was a general tendency toward normal lymphocyte counts in patients who had normal carcinoembryonic antigen (CEA) levels and toward depressed lymphocyte counts in patients with elevated CEA levels in their small group of patients. Fourteen of 25 patients with normal CEA levels also had counts greater than 2,000 cells/mm^3, while only 14 of 21 patients with elevated CEAs had such counts ($p < 0.05$). There was an inverse correlation between the preoperative CEA and lymphocyte levels in patients wth colorectal cancer. Bone and Lauder have observed a correlation not only between the lymphocyte count and the extent of disease (low counts in advanced disease) in patients with rectal and colon cancer and other gastrointestinal cancers, but also between the lymphocyte count and 2,4-dinitrochlorobenzene (DNCB) responses (21). Patients with low peripheral lymphocyte counts tended to have more advanced tumors and a poorer response to DNCB. Patients with colorectal cancer have been reported by Seitanides and Georgoulis to have not only depressed lymphocyte counts but also depressed T-cell levels (decreased numbers of rosette-forming lymphocytes) (22). The rosette inhibition test using antithymocyte globulin has been suggested to be an important indicator of T-cell competence, more so than the T-cell level or blastogenic response, in a study of colorectal-cancer patients by Ichiki et al (23).

DELAYED CUTANEOUS HYPERSENSITIVITY

Almost 50 years ago, Renaud first observed that tuberculin sensitivity was either depressed or absent in patients with malignant disease (24). In recent years, the value of measuring de novo hypersensitivity by using chemicals such as denitrofluorobenzene (DNFB) or DNCB has been well established (27–30). The DNCB reaction measures the gamut of the patient's immunologic response from initial antigen recognition (afferent limb) to final response (efferent limb). A correlation generally exists between a positive response to DNCB and a favorable prognosis following cancer surgery (28–30). Of particular importance in this type of study is the necessity of relating the immune responses to histologic type and stage of disease and to the recurrence and survival rates within each stage.

Patients with colorectal cancer have depressed skin-test responses to recall antigens. Kronman et al have found that patients with localized colorectal cancer and the control group responded similarly to recall antigens, but patients with regional nodal metastases show significantly depressed responses (31). DNCB reactivity in colorectal cancer has been measured by several authors (21,32–35). Bolton and Chakravorty et al demonstrated varying degrees of DNCB unreactivity in patients with localized colorectal cancer and marked depression in patients with metastatic disease (32,33).

Bone and Lauder found a statistically significant relationship between good DNCB responses and favorable pathologic stages, whereas a poor DNCB response correlated with an unfavorable stage (regional or distant metastases) (21). In our work (34,35), 237 patients with carcinoma of the colon and rectum and 16 patients with benign colorectal disease were skin-tested with DNCB and a battery of intradermal antigens (Table 2). The incidence of DNCB reactivity decreased with increasing stage of disease. Seventy-six percent of the patients with Dukes' A cancer were DNCB positive, compared to 56% of patients with Dukes' B lesions and 61% of patients with Dukes' C lesions. Of the patients with metastases beyond the bowel and its mesentery (usually the liver) at the time of primary surgery, 46% were DNCB positive. Only 42% of the patients with recurrent disease were responsive to DNCB; neither sex or age appeared to determine their response. Tumor burden appeared to correlate most closely with the patients's response to DNCB.

RELATION OF DELAYED
HYPERSENSITIVITY RESPONSES TO PROGNOSIS

At MSKCC, we have evaluated the relation of DNCB skin-test responses to short-term prognosis. Follow-up of 54 patients with Dukes' C cancer over 24 months showed a modest but not statistically significant improvement in recurrence rates in the DNCB-positive group. The disease recurred in 50% of 32 DNCB-positive patients, compared with 67% of 22 DNCB-negative patients (p = n.s). The relationship of DNCB to survival in patients with Dukes' C is not evaluable at this time, nor is the relationship to prognosis in Dukes' A or B patients yet established. Patients with advanced disease have not shown a significant relationship between DNCB response and survival.

IN VITRO TESTS OF IMMUNE REACTIVITY IN COLORECTAL CANCER*

Lymphocyte blastogenesis in response to mitogens has been the most frequently used of the in vitro tests of general cell-mediated immune reactivity, but the results have been variable. Lauder and Bone's 21 patients with colon cancer, as compared with 21 age-matched controls, showed a significant depression of dose–response curves with phyto-hemagglutinin-(PHA) (36). Similarly, Manousos et al found a significant reduction in the transformation of normal lymphocytes by PHA when they were cultured in the sera of cancer patients, as compared to lymphocytes cultured in control sera (37). The lymphocytes of some of the cancer patients were depressed even in the presence of control serum. Moreover, they discovered no relation of the blast transformation tests to the presence of lymph-node metastases. In contrast, Kaplan et al found no difference between controls and patients with both localized and metastatic colorectal cancer in the PHA response of lymphocytes cultured in the patients' serum (38). Similarly, Hsu and LoGerfo detected no statistical difference in the inhibitory effects of plasma in the colon-cancer and control patients (39). They did find a correlation of the plasma-inhibitory effect with the alpha globulin (the combined alpha-one and alpha-two globulins) (39). Goldrosen et al analyzed the lymphocyte blastogenic response in 76 colon-cancer patients and 29 age-matched controls and found both an age-related decline and a tumor-associated decline in immunocompetence in the cancer patients (40).

In our own study of lymphocyte blastogenesis as induced by mitogens in patients with colorectal cancer, we observed a depression in patients with Dukes' A lesions, a greater depression in patients with Dukes' B and C lesions (41), and maximum depression in patients with Stage IV lesions of recurrent disease (Table 2). We have not demonstrated a significant relationship of any of the in vitro tests to prognosis in patients with resectable Dukes' A, B, or C cancer. PHA-responsive lymphocyte levels

* See Table 1.

have correlated significantly with survival in patients with advanced cancer (41). This is contrasted with the prognostic relationship of CEA in which CEA level has significantly correlated with recurrence rates in patients with Dukes' B and C cancer (42). It has become obvious that no single test gives an adequate assessment of the immune reactivity in these patients. Possibly a profile consisting of many tests is more appropriate (43). Lurie et al studied an immunologic profile consisting of the circulating CEA, antigen-induced inhibition of mononuclear cell migration, skin reactivity to purified protein, streptokinase-streptodornase, and mumps, and tested this profile on 15 patients with colon cancer (43). Before surgery, 10 of 14 patients had elevated CEA, 12 of 12 showed a tumor-associated antigen-induced inhibition of mononuclear cell migration, and 10 of 11 failed to react to two or more recall antigens. Potential surgical cure in seven patients was accompanied by normal CEA in four, absent tumor-antigen–induced inhibition of mononuclear cell migration in all seven, and increased skin-test reactivity in six. Disseminated cancer in nine patients was associated with elevated CEA in all nine, absent mononuclear cell migration in seven, and suppressed skin reactivity in six of nine (43). A larger study group will be required to assess the true relevance of these results to prognosis in patients with colorectal cancer.

REACTIONS TO PUTATIVE TUMOR-ASSOCIATED ANTIGENS

The study of cell-mediated immune reactions to tumor cells is complex and controversial; for instance, the use of allogeneic test cells in many studies has produced a mass of confusing data and left the question of specificity unanswered. For this reason, we will concentrate on experience with cell-mediated responses to autologous tumor cells. Hellstrom et al, using the colony inhibition assay to study immunity against human colonic carcinoma, have found that colony formation of plated colon carcinoma cells was inhibited following the exposure to autochthonous lymphocytes from patients with colon cancer, and that this effect could be abrogated by serum, either autochthonous or allogeneic, from other patients with colon cancer (44–46). The same investigators, using the lymphocytotoxicity assay to demonstrate similar effects against colon-cancer cells, also found that, under certain conditions, serum from the cancer patient inhibited cytotoxicity of plated carcinoma cells by peripheral blood lymphocytes (47). These blocking factors seemed to represent either circulating tumor-specific antigen or circulating tumor-specific antibody and antigen complexes, but their precise nature remains unclear.

Nairn et al have conducted a large study of cell-mediated reactions to autochthonous colon-cancer cells (48). They studied 60 patients with colon cancer using short-term cultures of tumor cells and three assays: lymphocytotoxicity, complement-dependent serum cytotoxicity, and combined membrane and cytoplasmic immunofluorescence tests. Nineteen of the 60 patients responded positively to one or more tests. Lymphocytotoxicity was found in 8 of 24 patients, serum cytotoxicity was positive in 4 of 38, membrane fluorescence was positive in 7 of 55, and cytoplasmic fluorescence was positive in 10 of 59 patients. In a followup study made up, in part, of the same patient group, Piehl et al reported on lymphocytotoxicity studies of autochthonous cancer in 132 patients with colorectal cancer, in which they related the test results to stage, tumor differentiation, and absence of recurrence or metastatic spread (49). Peripheral blood lymphocytotoxicity was more common in patients with localized tumors (43%) than in those with metastases (17%) ($p < 0.01$). Positive tests occurred more frequently in patients with well-differentiated (64%) versus average or poorly differentiated tumors (25%). It is of interest that these investigators have also demonstrated that there is relative anergy of the lymphocytes residing within the cancer, as well as of the lymphocytes residing in the regional nodes, in comparison to the reactivity of the peripheral blood lymphocytes (17).

Nind et al found that none of the patients showed cytotoxic activity in the lymphocytes adjacent to the autologous cancer cells in ten patients with colon cancer, although there was cytotoxic activity in the peripheral blood lymphocytes in five patients. They also found that, although one-third (15 of 44 patients) of their colon-cancer patients had lymphocytotoxicity to autologous tumor cells in peripheral blood lymphocytes, only 1 of 33 patients had similar activity in the nodal lymphocytes (50). The same group also demonstrated serum inhibition of autochthonous lymphocytotoxicity in about 20% of the colon-cancer cases (50). The meaning of these studies remains to be clarified, but the results may be secondary to inhibition from circulating soluble antigens or antigen–antibody complexes. Of possible relevance here is the demonstration by Baldwin et al that papain-solubilized tumor-membrane extracts of pooled colon cancer inhibit cytotoxicity by sensitized lymphocytes against cultured colon-cancer cells, whereas extracts of normal colon or melanoma had no inhibitory effect (51). This would suggest that antigen exerts the inhibitory effect.

The above assays have depended on cultured tumor cells. Because of the major difficulties in obtaining even short-term cultured colon-cancer lines, the use of other assays, not dependent on tissue-culture lines, has been attempted. One such assay is the leukocyte migration-inhibition test (52), which has previously been used in studies of autologous primary breast cancer (53,54). Elias and Elias, using the leukocyte migration-inhibition test to study the response to autologous colon cancer in 48 patients with colorectal cancer, found that only patients with Dukes' C cancer showed a significant sensitization to their tumors (55). The peripheral blood leukocytes of these patients were sensitized to autologous tumor cells, but not to homologous tumor cells or normal colon tissue. House et al, using the same approach to study 31 patients with colorectal cancer, found that one-half of these patients showed 30% inhibition at some time in their postoperative period (56). These reactions were not related to the clinical or pathologic stage of the disease and varied among the patients, being transient in some and persistent in others. In addition, a positive response at a fixed time after operation was not found.

There have been several additional studies using the leukocyte migration inhibition test with homologous colon-cancer antigen preparations (57–60). Bull et al found a significant response to a mixed mononuclear cell migration inhibition test in the presence of the patient's leukocytes and allologous colon-cancer antigen (prepared as membrane-rich dilutions of homogenates of colon carcinomas) (57). Of 27 patients with operable colon cancer (Dukes' A, B, or C), 24 showed an inhibited migration response to the colon-cancer antigens. There was no inhibition of migration in any of the 52 cancer-free controls, nor in 9 patients who were surgically cured of adenocarcinoma of the colon (mean followup of 3.8 years). The clinical significance of this type of study is undetermined at this point. It may be that patients with operable cancer are actively sensitized to a common antigen as presented in the allologous tumor preparation, but that, following curative resection, this lymphocyte responsiveness is markedly diminished or lost. Other studies would suggest that such an antigen is not CEA, as CEA has not been shown to stimulate lymphocytes per se (61,62). Mavligit et al used lymphocyte blastogenesis to measure the immune response to autologous colon cancer obtained from right-sided colon lesions, and compared the response in the peripheral blood lymphocytes with that of lymphocytes obtained from the terminal ileum and the regional nodes (63). About 40% of the patients had positive responses in both the peripheral blood lymphocytes and the lymphocytes obtained from the terminal ileum, as compared to negative responses in the lymphocytes obtained from the regional lymph nodes (63).

Skin testing has also been used to demonstrate cell-mediated reactions to putative tumor-associated antigens in colon cancer. Hollinshead et al used soluble fractions from membranes of autologous colon-cancer cells in patients with carcinoma of the colon or rectum, discovering delayed hypersensitive responses to the cancer in 17 of 19 patients (64). They also demonstrated positive reactions to fetal gut extracts (64). By contrast, the response to similarly prepared fractions from normal cells of the colon was uniformly negative. Hollinshead also showed that, although there was CEA in the extracts used, the skin reactive component of these extracts was separate and distinct from purified CEA. Skin-test reactivity to purified CEA was not demonstrated (65).

HUMORAL IMMUNE RESPONSES TO COLON-CANCER ANTIGENS

In one of the earlier efforts to demonstrate humoral antibody responses to tumor-associated antigens of colon cancer in man, Hellstrom et al utilized tissue-culture lines of colon cancer and showed a cytotoxic antibody response (66). Schultz et al and Embleton et al have also demonstrated cytotoxic antibody to established cell lines of colon and rectal cancer (67,68). In Schultz's study, 8 of 14 patients with colon cancer had cytotoxic antibody to the cell line HCT-8, derived from a rectal cancer. In contrast, 12 of 15 patients with rectal cancer showed positive reactions to the rectal-cancer cell line as well as to the colonic-cancer cell line. The specificity of these reactions has not been rigidly defined. It is important to note that there have been some claims of humoral antibody responses in colon-cancer patients to purified CEA (69), but this has not been confirmed by other authors (70,71).

CARCINOEMBRYONIC ANTIGENS AND OTHER TUMOR MARKERS

Gold and Freedman initially described the carcinoembryonic antigen (CEA) as a colorectal cancer antigen that was tumor specific and was also a component of embryonic gut tissue (72), hence the derivation of the name. It was subsequently found that the antigen was present in normal adult colon tissue, although in much reduced amounts, and in normal serum, as well as in many other primary gastrointestinal malignancies (73–75). the carcinoembryonic antigen is a glycoprotein with a molecular weight of about 200,000 daltons, a sedimentation constant of 7–8 s, and 50 to 60% of carbohydrate-sialic acid, manose, galactose, acetylglucosamine, and fucose (71–78). The glycopeptide acetylglucosamine asparagine seems to be responsible for the greater part of the antigenic activity of CEA (79). CEA probably represents a family of heterogeneous molecules rather than a single molecule (80). We will not review here the extensive literature on CEA and would refer the reader to reviews by Burtin (71), Cooper et al (81), and Holyoke and Cooper (75). Thompson's demonstration that serum

Table 2. Relation of CEA to Stage of Disease in Colorectal Cancer*

Disease	Pts.	CEA Levels (ng/ml)			
		<5	5.1–10	10.1–20	>20
Benign colon lesions	47	100%			
Dukes' A	58	96%	4%		
Dukes' B	51	75%	11%	14%	
Dukes' C	63	55%	14%	13%	17%
Stage IV	31	35%	3%	19%	42%
Recurrent metastatic	155	28%	10%	16%	56%

* From Wanebo et al: *N Engl J Med* 299:449, 1978. (Used with permission.)

levels of CEA could be quantified by means of a radioimmunoassay led to the widespread and intensive study of this antigen and to the determination of its usefulness in patients with malignancy (82). Many studies have shown that CEA is not specific for colorectal cancer, and CEA elevations are found in other G.I. malignancies (83–86). CEA is frequently elevated in pancreatic cancer and gastric cancer with metastases, but it is elevated much less frequently in localized gastric cancer (86). CEA may also be elevated in benign disease such as inflammatory diseases of the bowel (75).

CEA has not been considered useful as a screening technique, but it may be useful as a diagnostic adjunct. McCartney and Hoffer found that although CEA was less specific and accurate than barium enema in diagnosing primary colon cancer, when both modalities were used simultaneously in their series of patients referred for barium enema, the percentage of detection rose from 65% with barium enema alone to over 90% when both modalities were used (87). Plasma CEA elevations probably reflect tumor burden, since the levels of CEA show a progressive increase with increasing stage of disease (88,89). In our own study of CEA levels in patients with primary colorectal cancer, the frequency of elevations increased with stage of disease. The percentages of patients showing elevations higher than the cutoff point of 5ng/ml were 5% in Dukes' A, 23% in Dukes' B, 38% in Dukes' C, and 56% in Stage IV (42) (Table 2). In patients with advanced disease CEA levels were highest with liver metastases and were much lower with local recurrence (Table 3).

CEA has also been reported to have prognostic usefulness. Herrera, et al (91) reported a series of 46 patients who underwent curative resection for colorectal cancer.

Table 3. Correlation of CEA Levels with Pattern of Recurrent Colorectal Cancer*

Metastatic Pattern	Pts.	<5 ng/ml	5.1–20 ng/ml	>20 ng/ml
Liver	52	8%	16%	76%
Lung–Bone	12	0	42%	58%
Abdomen–Viscera	45	36%	31%	33%
Local	46	50%	28%	22%
TOTAL	155	28%	26%	46%

* From Wanebo et al: *N Engl J Med* 299:450, 1978. (Used with permission.)

The mean preoperative CEA for those patients who later developed recurrence was 9.7 ng/ml compared to 2.15 ng/ml in the patients who did not recur. In their study of 23 patients who later developed recurrence, 19 had initial preoperative values greater than 2.5 ng/ml, and 4 had values above 4.0 ng/ml. In contrast, only 8 of 23 patients who did not demonstrate recurrence had values greater than 2.5 ng/ml, and only three had values above 4.0 ng/ml. Eight of 11 patients with Dukes' C lesions who subsequently developed recurrence had CEA values elevated above 2.5 ng/ml, compared to only one of the six patients who remained free of recurrence after 14 months (91). This would certainly suggest that CEA may yield prognostic information in addition to careful pathologic staging (91).

The experience with CEA on the Rectum and Colon Service at MSKCC has shown it to be of prognostic usefulness in patients with Dukes' B and C lesions (42). In either group there was a significant decrease in the disease-free interval in patients whose preoperative CEA was greater than 5 ng/ml. Other findings from this study have demonstrated that CEA levels are elevated in 92% of patients with liver metastases, but are elevated in only 50% of those with local recurrence. Moreover, the levels rise rapidly in patients with liver metastases whereas they are slow to rise in patients with local recurrence (42).

Probably the greatest usefulness of CEA will be in the detection of recurrence following curative resection of colorectal cancer. Neville and Cooper have summarized the literature dealing with this topic, and have tested 82 patients who developed recurrence and in whom CEA levels were monitored (91). In 19 patients there was no rise in CEA, whereas in 62 patients the CEA rose with or before recurrence. In 37 of these patients the CEA was reported as rising prior to clinical detection of recurrence (92). One must point out that there may be false positive elevations of CEA with subsequent return of these values to normal. There were 4 of 23 such patients in the Roswell Park series. Holyoke has suggested that three successive determinations be made ten days to two weeks apart in an attempt to confirm recurrence (75). If all these values are elevated above 2.5 ng/ml, and if they are rising, the patient faces approximately a 90% chance of recurrence of the disease. Certainly elevations above 5 ng/ml or single values greater than 25 ng/ml are very strongly suggestive of recurrence.

Martin et al have suggested that serial CEA determinations may provide information leading to a second-look procedure in patients who develop elevations of CEA after the normal postoperative drop (92). The authors have reported 22 patients who were reexplored, primarily because of elevations in the CEA, for possible recurrent colorectal cancer following an initial curative resection. In this study Martin and coworkers established a normogram and baseline in individual patients following a curative resection. If the CEA began to rise above the baseline and if there were two consecutive elevations in one month greater than 40% over the baseline, the investigators established new baseline values and repeated the study. If there were progressive increases for two consecutive months, they recommended a selected second-look procedure. Of 22 patients who were reexplored, all but three had elevated titers (these had shown progressive increases in titers using the normogram approach). Two of the three patients who had lung nodules were explored and found to have benign disease. Of 20 patients with abdominal exploration, all but one had recurrence. Ten of the 19 patients with recurrence had lesions resectable for cure. This type of study shows most clearly the potential benefit of CEA in salvaging patients in whom recurrence would otherwise have been missed, or operation delayed until the lesion was unresectable (93).

In preliminary data from the Rectum and Colon Service (MSKCC), there were 16 patients hospitalized for exploration because of CEA alone (93). Five patients had liver metastases, one had lung and liver metastases, one had lung metastases only, seven had local recurrence and two had negative laporatomies (one of these later succumbed to metastases). Although seven patients had lesions resected for cure, currently only four patients are alive and free of disease. This may reflect some delay in awareness or a delay in acting because of CEA elevation (all but one patient had CEA greater than 20 ng/ml at the time of exploration) (93). The true usefulness of this test in gaining patient salvage remains to be established.

The CEA may also provide a useful monitor of palliative therapy. Herera et al have reported a series of 75 patients with metastatic colon cancer receiving chemotherapy with 5-FU (94). There were 29 patients who showed a fall of CEA during treatment and 8 of these had a clearcut measurable response greater than 50%. Five of these eight patients were alive at the time of the report. Of the 21 patients who exhibited a fall in CEA but no clearcut clinical regression, 11 were still alive. In contrast, only 6 of 46 patients whose CEA values did not respond favorably to therapy were still alive (95). Although there is not yet a significant difference in the survival time of the CEA responders versus that of the CEA nonresponders, this study suggests a promising role for CEA as a monitor and possible prognostic indicator in patients receiving palliative therapy.

There are other markers besides CEA which have potential usefulness for monitoring patients with colorectal cancer. High on the list are enzyme markers of liver function changes and various serum protein functions. The reader is referred to reviews by Neville and Cooper (91), Cooper et al (95), Holyoke and Cooper (75) and Schwartz (96).

SUMMARY

We have reviewed some of the basic factors known to be involved in the immunobiology of colorectal cancer. From the morphologic point of view there is evidence of an immune response (or lack of it) in the primary cancer and in the regional nodes draining the cancer. General immune reactivity is frequently depressed, even in localized massive colorectal cancer, and becomes commonly depressed in patients with operable disease and regional node metastases or distinct metastases. Specific immune responses to putative tumor-associated antigens have been demonstrated by some authors, but not by others, and this field continues to be confused by an array of reports that discuss a multiplicity of assays but not a uniformity of reproducible results. One assay of a tumor marker, CEA stands out in its potential clinical usefulness. Although CEA is not specific for colorectal cancer (or any cancer per se), it is highly useful for postoperative monitoring of patients who have had curative resection of colorectal cancer. In some patients, postoperative CEA elevations have been the first evidence of recurrence.

We have reviewed a number of other immunological tests besides CEA and discussed the possible clinical utility of each one in patients with colon cancer. The question to ask each time is whether the test gives information that is useful in (1) detecting the presence of tumor, (2) estimating stage or extent of disease, (3) assigning prognosis, and/or (4) detecting recurrence. For each of the tests there have been some studies suggesting their usefulness, but in many cases, these have been balanced by studies that fail to confirm utility. Although this area of study is still in its infancy, there has been an explosion of immunologic data in recent years and newer, more sophisticated assays are being developed that may provide more relevant information about the immunobiology of colorectal cancer. There is already sufficient information to suggest that one or more of the currently used assays may find a place in the conventional, as well as the investigative, management of patients with colorectal carcinoma.

REFERENCES

1. The reader is referred to reviews collected in Good RA, Fisher DW (eds): *Immunobiology*. Stamford, Conn, Sinauer Assoc, 1973. Chap 1: Good RA, Disorders of the immune system. Chaps 3: Waksman B, Delayed hypersensitivity, immunologic and clinical aspects. Chap 10: Gewurz H, Immunologic role of complement. Chap 21: Hellstrom KE, Hellstrom F, Immunologic defenses against cancer.

2. Day NB, Good RA: Biological amplification systems in immunology, in Day NK, Good, RA (eds): *Comprehensive Immunology*. New York, Plenum, 1977, vol II.

3. Parrott DMV: The response of draining lymph nodes to immunological stimulation in intact and thymectomized animals. *J Clin Path* 20:456–465, 1967.

4. Parrott DMV, DeSousa MAB, East J: Thymus dependent areas in lymphoid organs of neonatally thymectomized mice. *J Clin Path* 20: 456–465, 1967.

5. Feldman M, Nossal CJV: Cellular bases of antibody production *Q Rev Biol* 47:269–302, 1972.

6. Mitchell GF, Miller JFAP: Cell to cell interactions in the immune response. *J Exp Med* 128:821, 1968.

7. Nossal GJV, Cunningham A, Mitchell GF, Miller JFAP: Cell to cell interaction in the immune response—III. Chromosomal marker analysis of single antibody forming cells in reconstituted irradiated and thymectomized mice. *J Exp Med* 128:839–854, 1968.

8. Andre JA, Schwartz RS, Metres WT, Dameshek W: The morphologic response of the lymphoid systems to homografts. *Blood* 19:313–333, 1962.

9. Edwards JA, Summer MR, Rowlands GF, Hard CM: Changes in lymphoreticular tissues during growth of a murine adenocarcinoma I. *J Natl Cancer Inst* 47:301–311, 1971.

10. Black MM, Kerpe S, Speer FD: Lymph node structure in patients with cancer of the breast. *Amer J Path* 29:505, 1953.

11. Black MM: Reactivity of LRE system in human cancer. *Prog Clin Cancer* 1:26–49, 1965.

12. Patt DJ, Byrnes RK, Vardiner JW, Coppelson LW: Mesocolic lymph node histology as an important prognostic indicator for patients with carcinoma of the sigmoid colon: an immunomorphologic study. *Cancer* 35:1388–1397, 1975.

13. Tsakraklides VT, Wanebo HJ, Sternberg S, et al: Prognostic evaluation of lymph node morphology in colorectal cancer. *Am J Surg* 129:174–180, 1975.

14. MacCarty WC, Mahle AE: Relation of differentiation and lymphocytic infiltration to postoperative survival in gastric carcinoma. *J Lab Clin Med* 6:473, 1921.

15. Moore OS, Foote FW Jr: The relatively favorable prognosis of medullary carcinoma of the breast. *Cancer* 2:635, 1949.

16. Sion A, Friedell M: Cellular immunity: polyps and carcinoma of the colon. *Int J Surg* 57:384, 1972.

17. Nind AP, Nairn RC, Rolland JM, et al: Lymphocyte anergy in patients with carcinoma. *Br J Cancer* 28:108–117, 1973.

18. Pihl E, Malahy MA, Khakhanian N, et al: Immunomorphological features of prognostic significance in Dukes' Class B colorectal carcinoma. *Cancer Res* 37:4145–4149, 1977.

19. Riesco A: Five year cure: relation to total amount of peripheral lymphocytes and neutrophils. *Cancer* 25:135–140, 1970.

20. Kim US: Lymphocyte counts in colon cancer patients. *J Surg Oncol* 8:257–262, 1976.

21. Bone G, Lauder I: Cellular immunity, peripheral blood lymphocyte counts and pathological staging of tumors in the gastrointestinal tract. *Br J Cancer* 30:215, 1974.

22. Seitanides B, Georgoulis G: Rosette forming lymphocyte counts in cancer of the colon, letter to the editor. *Lancet* 1:461, 1975.

23. Ichiki AT, Collmann IR, Sonoda T, et al: Inhibition of rosette formation by antithymocyte globulin: an indicator for T cell competence in colorectal cancer patients. *Cancer Immunol Immunother* 3:119–124, 1977.

24. Renaud M: La Cuti reaction a la tuberculin chez les cancereux. *Bull Soc Med Paris* 50:1441–1442, 1926.

25. Graham JB, Graham RM: Tolerance agent in human cancer. *Surg Gynecol Obstet* 118:1217–1222, 1964.

26. Hughes LE, McKay WD: Suppression of the tuberculin response in malignant disease. *Br Med J* 2:1346–1348, 1964.

27. Levin AG, McDonough EF, Miller DG, Southam CM: Delayed hypersensitivity responses in sick and healthy persons. *Ann N Y Acad Sci* 120:400, 1964.

28. Eilber FR, Morton DL: Impaired immunologic reactivity and recurrence following cancer surgery. *Cancer* 25:362–267, 1970.

29. Pinsky CM, Caron AS, Knapper WH, Oettgen HF: Delayed hypersensitivity in patients with cancer. *Proc Am Assoc Cancer Res* 12:399, 1971.

30. Pinsky CM, El Domieri AE, Caron AS, et al: Delayed hypersensitivity in patients with cancer. *Recent Results Cancer Res* 47:37–41, 1974.

31. Kronman BS, Shapiro HM, Localio SA: Delayed hypersensitivity responses of patients with carcinoma of the colon and other related tumors. *Dis Colon Rectum* 15(2):106–110, 1972.

32. Chakravorty RC, Cturchel HP, Coppalla PS, et al: The delayed hypersensitivity reaction in the cancer patient: observation or sensitization by DNCB. *Surgery* 73:730–735, 1973.

33. Bolton PM, Manda AM, Davidson JM, et al: Cellular immunity in cancer: comparison of delayed hypersensitivity skin tests in three common cancers. *Brit Med J* 3:18–20, 1975.

34. Rao B, Wanebo HJ, Pinsky CM, Stearns MW Jr, Oettgen HF: Delayed hypersensitivity reactions in colorectal cancer. *Surg Gynecol Obstet* 144:677–681, 1977.

35. Wanebo HJ, Rao B, Pinsky C, Stearns MW Jr, Oettgen HF, et al: Delayed hypersensitivity reactions in patients with colorectal cancer, in Crispen R (ed): *Neoplasm immunity: Mechanisms.* Chicago, ITR Publishers, 1976, pp 157–166.

36. Lauder I, Bone G: Lymphocyte transformation in large bowel cancer. *Br J Cancer* 28(1):78–79, 1973.

37. Manousos ON, Economou J, Pathouli CH, et al: Disturbance of cell mediated immunity in patients with carcinoma of colon and rectum. *Gut* 14:739–742, 1973.

38. Kaplan MS, Mino FO, Summerfeld KB, Lundak RL: Phytohemagglutinin-stimulated immune response. *Arch Surg* 110:1217–1220, 1975.

39. Hsu C, LoGerfo P: Correlation between serum alpha-globulin and the plasma inhibitory effects on PHA-stimulated lymphocytes in colon cancer patients *S E Biol Med* 139:575–578, 1972.

40. Goldrosen HH, Han T, Jung O, et al: Impaired lymphocyte blastogenic response in patients with colon adenocarcinoma: Effects of disease and age. *J Surg Oncol* 9:229–234, 1977.

41. Wanebo HJ, Rao B, Pinsky C, et al: Immunobiology of operable colorectal cancer. *Cancer* (in press).

42. Wanebo HJ, Rao B, Pinsky CM, et al: Preoperative carcinoembryonic antigen levels as a prognostic indicator in colorectal cancer. *N Engl J Med* 299:448–451, 1978.

43. Lurie BB, Bull D, Zamcheck N, et al: Diagnosis and prognosis in colon cancer based on profile of immune reactivity. *J Natl Cancer Inst* 54:319–325, 1975.

44. Hellstrom I, Hellstrom KE, Pearce GE, Yang JP: Cellular immunity to colonic carcinomas in man, in Burdette WJ (ed): *Carcinoma of the Colon and Antecedent Epithelium.* Springfield, Ill, Charles C Thomas, 1970, pp 176–188.

45. Hellstrom I, Hellstrom K, Shepard T: Cell mediated immunity against antigens common to human colonic carcinomas and fetal gut epithelium. *Int J Cancer* 6:346–351, 1970.

46. Hellstrom I, Hellstrom K, Sjogren H, Warner G: Demonstration of cell-mediated immunity to human neoplasms of various histologic types. *Int J Cancer* 7:1–16, 1971.

47. Hellstrom I, Hellstrom E et al: Newer concepts of cancer of the colon and rectum: Cellular immunity to human colonic carcinomas. *Dis Colon Rectum* 15(2):100–105, 1972.

48. Nairn RC, Nind AP, Guli EP, et al: Immunological reactivity in patients with carcinoma of the colon. *Br Med J* 4:706–709, 1971.

49. Piehl E, Hughes ES, Nind AP, Nairn RC: Colonic carcinoma: clinicopathological correlation with immunoreactivity. *Br Med J* 3:742–743, 1975.

50. Nind AP, Matthews N, Piehl EA, et al: Analysis of serum inhibition of lymphocyte cytotoxicity in human colon carcinoma. *Br J Cancer* 31:620–629, 1975.

51. Baldwin RW, Embleton MJ, Price MR: Inhibition of lymphocyte cytotoxicity for human colon carcinoma by treatment with solubilized tumour membrane fractions. *Int J Cancer* 12(1):84–92, 1973.

52. Soborg M, Bendixen G: Human lymphocyte migration as a parameter of hypersensitivity. *Acta Med Scand* 181:247–256, 1967.

53. Anderson V, Bendixen G, Schiodt T: An in vitro demonstration of cellular immunity against autologous mammary cancer in man. *Acta Med Scand* 186:101, 1969.

54. Segall A, Weiler O, Gevin J, Lacour F: In vitro study of cellular immunity against autochthonous human cancer. *Int J Cancer* 9:417, 1972.

55. Elias E, Elias L: Some immunologic characteristics of carcinoma of the colon and rectum. *Surg Gynecol Obstet* 141:715–718, 1975.

56. House AK, Wisniewski S, Woodings B: Immunity in colonic tumor patients after operation. *Dis Colon Rectum* 18:100–106, 1975.

57. Bull D, Leibad JR, Williams MA, Helms RA: Immunity to colon cancer assessed by antigen-induced inhibition of mixed mononuclear cell migration. *Science* 181:957–959, 1973.

58. Armistead PR, Gowland G: The leukocyte adherence inhibition test in cancer of the large bowel. *Br J Cancer* 32:568–573, 1975.

59. Guillou PJ, Brennan TG, Giles GR: A study of lymph nodes draining colorectal cancer using a two stage inhibition of leukocyte migration technique. *Gut* 16:290–297, 1975.

60. Maluish A, Halliday WJ: Cell mediated immunity and specific serum factors in human cancer: The leukocyte adherence inhibition test. *J Natl Cancer Inst* 52:1415, 1975.

61. Lejtenyi MC, Freedman SO, Gold P: Response of lymphocytes from patients with gastrointestinal cancer to the carcinoembryonic antigen of the human digestive system. *Cancer* 285:120, 1971.

62. Strauss E, Vernace T, Janowitz H, Paronetto F: Migration of peripheral leukocytes in the presence of carcinoembryonic antigen. *Proc Soc Biol Med* 148:494–497, 1975.

63. Mavligit GM, Jubet AV, Gutterman JV, et al: Immune reactivity of lymphoid tissues adjacent to carcinoma of the ascending colon. *Surg Gynecol Obstet* 139:409–412, 1974.

64. Hollinshead A, Glew D, Bunnag B, et al: Skin-reactive soluble antigen from intestinal cancer-cell-membranes and relationship to carcinoembryonic antigens. *Lancet* 1:1191–1195, 1970.

65. Hollinshead AC, McWright CG, Alford TC, et al: Separation of skin reactive intestinal cancer antigen from the carcinoembryonic antigen of Gold. *Science* 177:887–889, 1972.

66. Hellstrom I, Hellstrom KE, Pierce GE, Yang JP: Cellular and humoral immunity to different types of human neoplasms. *Nature* 220:1352–1354, 1968.

67. Schultz RM, Woods WA, Cherigos MA: Detection in colorectal carcinoma patients of antibody cytotoxicity to established cell strains derived from carcinoma of the human colon and rectum. *Int J Cancer* 16:16–23, 1975.

68. Embleton MJ, Price MR: Inhibition of cell mediated cytotoxicity against human colon carcinomatic by papain-solubilized tumour membrane extracts. *Br J Cancer* 28:148–152, 1973.

69. Gold P: Circulating antibodies against carcinoembryonic antigens of the human digestive system. *Cancer* 20:1663–1667, 1967.

70. LoGergo P, Herten F, Bennett S: Absence of circulatory antibodies of carcinoembryonic antigen in patients with gastrointestinal malignancies. *Int J Cancer* 9:344–348, 1972.

71. Burtin P: Membrane antigens of colonic tumors. *Cancer* 34:829–832, 1974.

72. Gold P, Freedman SO: Specific carcinoembryonic antigens of the human digestive system. *J Exp Med* 127:467–481, 1965.

73. Chu TM, Reynoso G, Hansen HJ: Demonstration of carcinoembryonic antigen in normal human plasma. *Nature* 238:152–153, 1972.

74. Burtin P, Von Kleist S, Chanonel G: Further studies on carcinoembryonic antigen. NIC, Monographs 35:421–425, 1972.

75. Holyoke ED, Cooper EH: CEA and tumor markers. *Semin Oncol* 4:377–385, 1976.

76. Banjo C, Gold P, Freedman JO, Krupey J: Immunologically active heterosaccharides of carcinoembryonic antigen of human digestive system. *Nature* 238:183–185, 1972.

78. Krupey J, Gold P, Freedman SO: Physiochemical studies of the carcinoembryonic antigens of the human digestive system. *J Exp Med* 128:387–398, 1968.

79. Banjo C, Gold P, Freedman SO, Krupey J: Structure of the immunodominant tumor grouping of CEA of the human. *Fed Proc* 32:1007, 1973.

80. Coligan JE, Henkact PA, Todd CW, and Terry WD: Heterogeneity of the carcinoembryonic antigen. *Immunochemistry* 10:591–600, 1973.

81. Cooper EH, Turner R, Steele L, et al: The contribution of serum enzymes and CEA to the early diagnosis of metastatic colorectal cancer. *Br J Cancer* 31:111–117, 1975.

82. Thompson DMP, Krupey J, Freedman SO, et al: The radioimmunoassay of circulating carcinoembryonic antigens of the digestive system. *Proc Natl Acad Sci USA* 64:161, 1969.

83. LoGerfo P, Krupey J, Hansen J: Demonstration of an antigen common to several varieties of neoplasia: Assay using zirconyl phosphate gel. *N Engl J Med* 285:138, 1971.

84. Reynoso G, Chu TM, Holyoke ED, et al: Carcinoembryonic antigen in patients with different cancers. *JAMA* 220:361–365, 1972.

85. Lawrence DJR, Stevens U, Bettelheim R, et al: Role of plasma carcinoembryonic antigen in diagnosis of gastrointestinal, mammary and bronchial carcinoma. *Br Med J* 3:605–609, 1972.

86. Ravry M, McIntire KR, Moertel CG, et al: Carcinoembryonic antigen and alpha-fetoprotein in the diagnosis of gastric and colonic cancer; a comparative clinical evaluation. *J Natl Cancer Inst* 152:1019–1021, 1974.

87. McCartney WH, Hoffer PB: The value of carcinoembryonic antigen (CEA) as an adjunct to the radiological colon examination in the diagnosis of malignancy. *Radiology* 110:325–328, 1974.

88. Dhar P, Moore T, Zamcheck N, et al: Carcinoembryonic antigen (CEA) in colonic cancer. *JAMA* 221:31–35, 1972.

89. LoGerfo P, LoGerfo F, Herter F, et al: Tumor associated antigens in patients with cancer of the colon. *Am J Surg* 123:127–131, 1972.

90. Herrera M, Chu TM, Holyoke ED: Carcinoembryonic antigen (CEA) as a prognostic and monitoring test in clinically complete resection of colorectal carcinoma. *Ann Surg* 183:509, 1976.

91. Neville SM, Cooper EH: Biochemical monitoring of cancer. *Ann Biochem* 13:283–305, 1976.

92. Martin EW, James KK, Hurtubise PE, et al: The use of CEA as an early indication for gastrointestinal tumor recurrence and second look procedure. *Cancer* 39:440–446, 1977.

93. Wanebo HJ, Stearns MW Jr, Schwartz MK: Use of CEA as an indicator of early recurrence and as a guide to a selected second-look procedure in patients with colorectal cancer. *Ann Surg* 188:481–493, 1978.

94. Herrera M, Chu TM, Holyoke ED, et al: CEA monitoring of palliative treatment for colorectal cancer. *Ann Surg* 185:23–30, 1977.

95. Cooper EH, Turner R, Steee L, et al: The contribution of serum enzymes and CEA to early diagnosis of metastatic colorectal cancer. *Br J Cancer* 31:111–117, 1975.

96. Schwartz M: An evaluation of markers in the early detection of large bowel cancer. *Cancer* 40:2620–2624, 1977.

13
The Care
of the Patient
with a Colostomy

Maus W. Stearns, Jr.

INTRODUCTION

The rehabilitation of a patient with a colostomy varies with the type and location of the colostomy, whether or not the patient is free of cancer, and the physical and mental ability of the patient to cope with the mechanics of colostomy care. These factors are compounded by the attitudes of the patients and their families toward the colostomy, which in turn are conditioned by varying ethnic and social backgrounds and previous experiences they may have had with colostomies in varying degrees of control and acceptability. With a full understanding and adaptation to these preconditions, the vast majority of patients who have had a colostomy performed in the course of a curative resection for cancer of the rectum can and do live useful, functional lives. They must receive competent, knowledgeable, and sympathetic instruction in the details of the management of their colostomy and have the support of their family and physician.

TYPES OF COLOSTOMIES

Curative or Palliative

The basic cancer pathological process for which a colostomy is performed is a major factor influencing the ability of the patient to make a satisfactory adjustment. If the colostomy is performed in the course of a curative operation, the problems of adjustment are mechanical and psychological. If, however, a colostomy is performed for an inoperable tumor, then the problems of adjusting to the colostomy are of minor importance as compared to the problems of the cancer.

Patients who are extremely resistant to a needed colostomy often have had previous unpleasant experiences with other patients who had colostomies performed for palliation. Their concepts of the problems of a colostomy are more often those of terminal cancer symptoms rather than those of a colostomy per se.

Temporary or Permanent

Temporary colostomies for cancer are most often performed with anterior resection of rectosigmoid carcinoma to provide protection while the anastomosis heals. They may be performed also as emergencies for relief of obstruction in various portions of the large bowel, most often of the left colon. Permanent colostomies most frequently are performed in the course of abdominoperineal resection for cancer of the rectum, resulting in sigmoid or left-sided colostomies.

Temporary colostomies by virtue of their limited duration seldom cause the problems one sees with a permanent colostomy, primarily because the patient, knowing the limited duration of the colostomy, accepts the handicaps more readily. On the other hand, the knowledge that one has to live with a permanent colostomy the rest of one's life compounds the mechanical and other psychologic problems the patient has to meet.

Physiologic Location of Colostomy

Since the primary function of the colon is water absorption, the location within the colon of the colostomy is a significant factor in its management. The bowel content of the right colon is liquid and enters the colon more or less continuously from the small bowel. While there may be some physiologic adaptation of the terminal ileum to increase water absorption, this is never complete, and the stool consistency remains that of a thick liquid expelled frequently. To collect this liquid, more-or-less continuous evacuatant receptacles are necessary. To prevent skin irritation and spillage that soils the skin and clothing, the receptacles should adhere firmly to the skin.

In the more distal sigmoid sufficient water has been absorbed so that the bowel content is relatively solid, similar to the contents of the normal rectum. Because of its solid nature, the bowel content is not expelled continuously but is normally evacuated in a solid or soft solid state by the peristaltic rush of the colon several times a day. If appliances are used, they do not have to adhere to the skin. Also, the more solid state of the stool permits some degree of control by the use of irrigations to initiate the peristalsis that empties the left colon. This evacuation in most persons ensures freedom from further fecal expulsion from the colostomy for 48 hours, and occasionally longer. In some people this irrigation is effective for only 24 hours. In a few persons, it is completely ineffective, as they continue to have fecal spill irregularly throughout the day and night.

In the transverse colon the consistency of the bowel content is somewhere between the liquid of the ileum and the solid of the sigmoid. Usually the feces is so loose as to require a skin-adherent appliance as a receptacle. Also, in most people evacuation occurs so frequently that irrigations are not effective in initiating a single large evacuation that provides effective control for any substantial period of time. Thus in practice, the value of teaching any method of irrigations of a temporary transverse colostomy is equivocal.

INDICATIONS AND CONTRAINDICATIONS FOR COLOSTOMY

In view of the limited duration of the temporary colostomies, indications and contraindications are of less importance to the rehabilitation of the patient, since these colostomies will usually be closed within a matter of a few months at most. However, because each colostomy involves additional hospitalization and morbidity, the procedure should not be performed thoughtlessly or "routinely." In the past and also, to some extent, at this time, a number of permanent colostomies with their attendant problems have been and are being performed unnecessarily, in our opinion.

The most frequent and best established indication for a permanent colostomy is cancer of the mid and distal rectum, for which a sigmoid colostomy is formed as part of an abdominoperineal resection of the rectum. A Miles' type of abdominoperineal resection for clinically invasive cancer of the distal rectum is the only procedure that has proved its value in long-term survival for these patients. This statement is based on its wide use over many years, correlated with the results obtained, which are roughly 50% five-year survival throughout the United States. Furthermore, the only overall improvement in survival rates for patients with cancer of the rectum in the past 30 years has been directly related to increased resectability rates.

Contraindications to permanent colostomy in our opinion are real; some are quite specific while others are equivocal. A colostomy should not always be done for a nonobstructing rectal carcinoma in the presence of extensive liver, peritoneal, or pulmonary metastases. The unnecessary addition of a colostomy often adds more problems for the patient who is sick and debilitated from metastatic disease. The nonobstructing rectal lesion often can be reasonably well controlled by local means, such as local excision, fulguration, cryosurgery, or radiation therapy. However, abdominoperineal resection with permanent colostomy may well be the most effective way to bring relief to the patient with a tumor of the rectum that is obstructing or producing significant amounts of irritating bloody discharge, even though liver metastases are present.

The most abused contraindication to a permanent colostomy is the use of an abdominoperineal resection for tumors in such a location that equally good chances for five-year survival can be achieved by sphincter-preserving procedures, which avoid a permanent colostomy. In general, the majority of cancers of the upper rectum and distal sigmoid, that is, above 7–8 cm from the anal verge, can be treated just as well by sphincter-preserving operations, particularly anterior resections, as by Miles' type of abdominoperineal resections.

MECHANICAL CONSIDERATIONS OF COLOSTOMY

Principles of Construction

Colostomies should be constructed to achieve the following desirable characteristics in the matured stoma:

1. Slight protrusion of the stomal mucosa above the skin level about a quarter inch
2. An adequate but not patulous stomal lumen that admits the little finger snugly
3. The location should be such that it is easily visualized and readily accessible for care; that it should not interfere with belts, nor be subject to trauma from occupational habits such as leaning against benches; that it can easily be kept clean—thus it should not be immediately adjacent to the umbilicus or in a roll of fat.
4. The descending and sigmoid colon should be brought out to the abdominal wall from

its peritoneal attachment with a gentle curve, leaving no redundant loops below the abdominal wall to angulate or obstruct elimination or irrigations.

These characteristics can be achieved in a number of ways. Our particular approach at MSKCC entails mobilizing the sigmoid colon sufficiently to eliminate any redundant loops or curves, bringing the colon out through the operative incision (a left paramedian) about 2 inches below the umbilicus, and closing the abdominal wall about it tightly enough to allow only the introduction of the little finger along the antimesenteric border. We use no sutures within the abdominal cavity. We do not mature the colostomy primarily. We place a necrosing clamp across the bowel about one fingerbreadth above the skin for 48 hours. If at the end of seven to eight days the protruding colon is larger than a fingerbreadth, we amputate the excess, using a scalpel and cautery to control bleeding.

Limitations Imposed by Colostomy

With a well-constructed colostomy that is properly located, without redundant protruding bowel and without a pericolostomy hernia, there are no limitations to physical activity, with the possible exception of very heavy lifting or straining. Normal moderate exercises are tolerated and are desirable. Showering, bathing, and swimming should be encouraged. The resection of the rectum and establishment of the colostomy do not weaken the body in any way, as is imagined by many patients.

The only major handicap associated with a well-constructed colostomy is the removal of sphincteric control, with loss of ability to retain flatus and feces. This loss of voluntary control of fecal discharge is a source of great emotional disturbance to patients, not only because they may be soiled with fecal material when it is inconvenient to cleanse themselves or under embarrassing circumstances, but also because they feel that they are no longer able to meet a minimum social requirement of our society, that is, control of fecal evacuation.

Irrigations of Colostomy

In an effort to restore some degree of control of bowel movement, not only for the patient's convenience, but also to restore some sense of being able to control the time and place of fecal evacuation, we have used mechanical irrigations as a substitute for sphincteric control. Most patients, after being properly taught a method of irrigation and learning to avoid the particular foods that cause them diarrhea, are able to irrigate every 48 h and remain free of fecal soilage between irrigations.

There are many methods of irrigation, each with advantages and disadvantages. We had for many years used a closed method using the Binkley-Deddish Colostomy Irrigation set. There are many very acceptable modifications that retain the same principles. One of these is an appliance that fits over the colostomy and is held in place by a belt. In the middle of the appliance is an opening through which an irrigating catheter can be passed. The appliance is connected to a plastic sheath, through which the fecal return is led into the toilet bowel. The irrigating catheter is attached by tubing to a rubber bag which holds a quart of water. This bag is suspended so that its lower level is at the level of the patient's shoulder. The irrigating bag is filled with lukewarm tap water.

Air is removed from the tubing and irrigating catheter by running water through them. The flow of water is controlled by a clamp. The catheter is well lubricated, passed through the opening in the center of the appliance and introduced into the colostomy 3 to 4 inches. The water is then allowed to run into the colostomy slowly. (Speed is regulated by the height of the bag.) The flow is interrupted if the patient has any feeling of distention, cramps, or discomfort. The irrigation catheter is then withdrawn. The patient remains on the commode with the plastic sheath in the bowl until the water and fecal contents is expelled. This may require 30 to 60 min. For the first month or so it is advisable for the patient to then close the plastic sheath by folding it over and fastening it with a clamp or rubber band. He may then move about, performing some simple activity such as shaving, while the cup and sheath is in place for an hour or so as there may be additional discharge after the initial evacuation.

On completion of the irrigation the patient then puts a piece of gauze, well lubricated with vaseline, directly over the colostomy, with a heavier absorbent pad on top held in place by a girdle, or a man's supportive belt, such as a girdle or wide-band athletic supporter, or a special surgical belt. The pad usually requires daily change if only for the mucus that seeps out.

Problems with Irrigations

The most common problem associated with irrigation is the prolonged time required for a satisfactory evacuation. Usually this is due to constipation and should be corrected by dietary means or mild laxatives. Irrigating time may sometimes be speeded by using mildly soapy water instead of plain tap water. Difficulty in inserting the catheter in a properly constructed colostomy without angles or kinks or paracolostomy hernias is almost always due to the presence of constipated stool.

Loss of irrigating fluid, that is, irrigating water that comes out around the catheter while being introduced, most frequently results from hard inspissated feces blocking the inflow of water. If this is a constant problem, some retaining device may be used. Several very simple methods are effective. A nipple from a baby's bottle with a hole in the nipple large enough to allow the catheter to pass through, held firmly against the stoma to retain the water, is inexpensive and effective. A rubber ear syringe or rubber ball may be used in the same way. Graduated Laird cones are very useful.

Appliances

A number of surgeons do not like the method of irrigation and do not advise their patients to use it. A few patients, after they have been taught the method of irrigation, feel that it is not worth the effort. Also, a few patients cannot develop a successful pattern of irrigation, having fecal discharge in spite of irrigation. For these patients a number of very satisfactory appliances are available. These appliances should have the following characteristics. They should be made of plastic, as rubber rapidly acquires an offensive odor that cannot be eliminated. The appliance should fit snuggly to the abdominal wall, being just slightly larger than the stoma itself, minimizing skin exposure. Usually it does not need to adhere to the skin, but it should not be so loose so that it abrasively rubs over the skin. Often Karaya rings on the inner surface of the appliance protect the skin and prevent irritation from bowel content. The belt holding the appliance in place should be such that it can easily be fastened by the patient and should be constructed and located so that it does not move up and down, shifting out of position.

Diet

One of the most widespread misconceptions is that patients with colostomies must be on a restricted, constipating diet. Actually, patients are able to manage their colostomies best if they take a well-rounded diet, including vegetables and fruit, both raw and cooked. The diet should be regulated to avoid either constipation from too little bulk or diarrhea from too much bulk. Most patients find a few specific foods are not tolerated. These are learned by trial and error.

Patients are advised to add to the basic hospital diet any food they like, one at a time with ample time to observe the effects before the next addition. They are warned that some foods may not be tolerated and should be experimented with carefully. Among these, which will be supplemented by individual idiosyncracies, are sauerkraut, corn, white or red beans, onions, highly spiced or seasoned foods, carbonated drinks, especially beer, milk, and iced drinks, particularly large amounts of ice water or iced tea.

Medications

Patients with colostomies may ordinarily take any medications they tolerated previously. However, some medications do cause hypermotility of the colon, which in an ostomate leads promtly to diarrhea. Hence, medication should be prescribed with care, and when diarrhea occurs, viewed with suspicion. The patient with a colostomy who is regularly constipated needs to be encouraged to ingest more bulk in the form of fruits and vegetables. When occasionally constipated, the patient may take laxatives; a combination of mineral oil and milk of magnesia in doses of 30 cc of each once or twice daily is very satisfactory.

The ostomate with occasional episodes of diarrhea should be warned to try to correlate these with ingested food or drink. If the diarrhea persists for more than 24 h, a diet of boiled milk, tea, and toast will often control it promptly. Kaopectate is a useful supplement. If diarrhea persists for more than two to three days, 45 cc of castor oil may be the most effective way of eliminating the responsible offender. The patient who has enjoyed regular bowel pattern after a colostomy for some months or years and then develops a definite change in bowel habit should be investigated for a new tumor or metastases.

Magnetic Colostomy

Considerable interest has been aroused concerning the subcutaneous implantation of a magnetic ring about a colostomy, which then holds a metallic cap over the colostomy. From early reports of actual experience with these devices, it is apparent that they are associated with technical problems and complications, which appear to be extensive enough to contraindicate their routine use at the present time. They may offer some help to the few patients who cannot learn to cope with their colostomies by the methods described.

PSYCHOLOGIC IMPACT OF COLOSTOMY

A number of basic articles have been written on the psychologic impact of a colostomy, the one by Sutherland, Orbach, Dyk, and Bard being most useful to us (2). The following concepts have been helpful in understanding a patient with a colostomy and have guided our efforts at rehabilitation.

On Patients

The most basic concern of a patient with a colostomy is the inability to control elimination of bowel content, which has been discussed earlier. Another psychologic problem is that many patients believe that removal of the rectum has caused irreparable harm to their bodies, that their body strength has been seriously impaired. Patients harboring these beliefs often complain of weakness and lack of strength years after they have recovered from their operations and are in good physical health. They need thorough explanations and constant reassurance that there has been no major loss of their ability to function.

Another major problem for patients is the basic fear of the cancer for which they were treated in the first place. While space does not permit a thorough discussion of the semantics of the word *cancer,* it often conjures up fears of a disease process that cannot be cured. Gentle probing as to what patients understand they had in the first place and what they believe their future to be are often very helpful, in at least partially easing this concern.

Manifestations of Nonacceptance of Colostomy

Patients who are unwilling to accept the fact of their colostomies and make the best of it seldom communicate this directly to the surgeon or their physician. However, the fact of unacceptance may be obvious to their families, who may, if given the opportunity, volunteer the observation of change in personality.

The patient's lack of acceptance may be manifested in other ways. The physically and mentally competent patient who is unable to manage the colostomy by any means, after real efforts at rehabilitation, in all likelihood has simply rejected the idea that it is possible to cope with it and refuses to try. Because the impact of the colostomy overshadows any of their other problems which might be helped by their physician, these patients refuse to return to the surgeon or physician, because the doctor could do nothing about eliminating the colostomy. They may then claim abandonment on the part of their physicians. Some feel so harmed both by the operation and the colostomy that they withdraw from society and never again perform any useful work, even though they are entirely competent to do so. These and other manifestations point to the conviction of such patients that they are socially unacceptable, physically impaired, and unable to lead any kind of useful lives. While our best efforts to convince them otherwise sometimes fail, much can be done if we recognize the basic problem and try to educate them as to their worth.

Affect on Family

Dyk and Sutherland have written an excellent review of this problem (1). In brief, they point out the many different types and qualities of preoperative relationships within families, all of which affect the postoperative reaction. In general, where relationships have been strong preoperatively they remain strong postoperatively, with the spouse giving support and real help in the early postoperative period. If the relationships have been poor or weak preoperatively, very little support or help can be expected postoperatively, and the poor quality of the relationship becomes worse. It is important to assess family relationships in our rehabilitative efforts. Sending patients who have many doubts and fears themselves to homes where there is an unaccepting environment will confirm their worse expectations and turn temporary concerns into permanent ones. Conversely, the same patient sent home to a warmly supportive family more easily regains confidence and resumes an essentially normal preoperative pattern of living.

CONCLUSIONS

The rehabilitation of the patient with a colostomy can usually be very satisfactory, providing the mechanical and psychologic aspects are understood and given appropriate attention.

REFERENCES

1. Dyk RB, Sutherland AM: Adaptation of the spouse and other family members to the colostomy patient. *Cancer* 9:123–138, 1956.
2. Sutherland AM, Orbach CE, Dyk RB, Bard M: The psychologic impact of cancer and cancer surgery. 1. Adaptation to the dry colostomy; preliminary report and summary of findings. *Cancer* 5:857–872, 1952.
3. Stearns MW Jr: The patient with a colostomy, in Schottenfeld, D (ed): *Cancer, Epidemiology and Prevention.* Springfield, Ill, Charles C Thomas, 1975.

14

Guidelines for the Follow-up of Patients with Carcinomas and Adenomas of the Colon and Rectum

Fadi F. Attiyeh

FOLLOW-UP OF PATIENTS WITH CARCINOMA OF THE COLON AND RECTUM

The case of the patient with carcinoma of the colon and rectum, like patients with cancer in any other organ, should be closely followed for life because of the risk of developing the following:

- Recurrence of disease, either local or systemic
- Metachronous lesions in the colon and rectum
- Other primary cancers in other organs

Tumor Recurrence

The cure rate for patients who have undergone resection of carcinoma of the colon and rectum reached its peak about two decades ago and has remained stationary ever since. In fact, about 50% of all patients with colorectal carcinoma who undergo "curative" resection will eventually develop recurrent cancer. Roughly half of these patients, particularly those with cancer of the rectum, develop local lesions, and the other half develop distant metastases. Most of the recurrences occur in the first two to three years after resection, and the risk decreases exponentially as time goes on; therefore, the follow-up should be at more frequent intervals during the critical early years, when recurrences are more likely to occur.

Local recurrent disease is usually beyond surgical cure, but there are many instances where survival, or palliation for a reasonable period of time, can be achieved, particularly if the recurrence is detected at an early stage. Early anastomotic recurrences and solitary liver and lung metastases may be resected with a good chance of cure. In our experience, the five-year survival rates for patients with resected solitary liver and lung metastases are 40% and 22%, respectively (1,2).

Metachronous Lesions in the Colon and Rectum

It appears true that if one area of the large-bowel mucosa develops a tumor, there is an increased chance that other portions of the mucosa, being continuously subjected to the insult of one or more factors that are presently largely unknown, which possibly caused the original tumor, will thus develop one or more additional lesions. In addition, there are some indications that the colonic mucosa at a distance from the tumor shows some abnormalities in the width and depth of the crypts, as well as some cellular changes on electron microscopy (3). The reported incidence of metachronous cancers in the colon and rectum varies between 2 and 6% (4,5). A review of our experience shows that the incidence curve is biphasic, with a peak during the first 4 to 5 years, and another after 10 to 12 years (5). The first peak probably represents the lesions that were truly synchronous in the form of an adenoma or an early carcinoma that went undetected and progressed to a clinically obvious cancer later on. That is why it is important to evaluate the large bowel carefully by either one or a combination of the following: barium enema, colonoscopy, and colotomy–coloscopy when the patient is being treated for a first primary cancer. In brief, the patient successfully treated for colon cancer should be diligently followed for life, in order to detect a second lesion at a premalignant or early stage and thereafter to achieve and maintain a disease-free state.

Other Primary Cancers in Other Organs

By the same token, as mentioned for the development of metachronous lesions, the patient with cancer of the large bowel has a higher risk of developing a cancer in another organ, notably the breast or lung (6,7). The immunologic system of the patient, as well as obscure tumor-host relationship and environmental factors that led to development of the first lesion, could well be instrumental in the development of another lesion in another organ. Since careful and close follow-up of the patient with cancer of the colon and rectum appears worthwhile, the following steps should be followed.

History

Paying attention to the patient's description of symptoms cannot be overemphasized. The patient who had been successfully treated for a tumor and is asymptomatic may develop any one or a combination of symptoms that should direct attention toward the possible occurrence of disease:

- Rectal bleeding may indicate an anastamotic recurrence or the development of a new tumor.
- A change in bowel habits and flatulence may similarly be indicative of recurrence or a new tumor.
- Abdominal cramps may signify impending obstruction, which in about half of the cases is due to recurrent disease.
- Pain in the upper abdomen, particularly the right upper quadrant radiating to the shoulder and back, suggests the possibility of liver metastasis.

- Perineal or pelvic pain, particularly if it radiates along the posterior thigh, following abdominoperineal resection and after a pain-free interval, is usually diagnostic of recurrent pelvic disease.
- The development of a cough, with or without hemoptysis, may signal the presence of lung metastasis or a new lung primary.
- Headaches or peripheral muscle weakness may signal brain or cord metastases.

Physical Examination

This should be done at each visit with more emphasis given to systems signalled by the particular symptoms of the patient. Of importance is the detection of any peripheral lymphadenopathy, skin nodules, abdominal masses, and so on. The rectal exam is a must at each visit; a low rectal anastamosis can be palpated for recurrence, new lesions in the anorectum can be ruled out, and pelvic recurrence can be assessed. Blood on the examining finger warrants additional search for the source. The pelvic examination should be periodically performed to detect any extension of tumor into the vagina. The parametria can be examined for the detection of ovarian masses.

Sigmoidoscopy should be performed at each visit for patients whose anastamosis is within reach of the sigmoidoscope. It should be done routinely twice a year in other patients, and if new symptoms warrant the procedure. Hemoccult slides by the Greegor method have proved to be quite valuable in the early detection of polyps and cancer (8). This procedure can also be helpful for the detection of early anastamotic recurrences. The test is quite simple and can be done with each visit. The patient should be on a meat-free diet for three days to minimize false positives.

Carcinoembryonic Antigen

The level of carcinoembryonic antigen has become one of the most significant markers in cancer of the colon and rectum. In several articles, a correlation between elevated carcinoembryonic antigen levels and the occurrence of recurrent disease is discussed (9–11). The test, however, should be evaluated carefully, in context with other serial determinations, particularly if a baseline level is obtained; a rise above previous levels is significant. The carcinoembryonic antigen level should be determined frequently in high-risk patients, at least every two to three months during the first two years. If a significant elevation is detected, it should be verified by repeating the test twice in a short period, and if the results are consistently high, further diagnostic workup is indicated to detect recurrence. In some instances a laparotomy may have to be performed, and in some cases localized recurrence can be resected to render the patient disease free (12,13).

Carcinoembryonic antigen determinations in colonic washings is a promising method for early detection of small mucosal lesions but is still in an experimental stage and probably is not practical for wide use.

Chest X-Ray Films

Simple posteroanterior and lateral films of the chest should be done at least every six months for the first three to four years and yearly afterward, in any patient with cancer of the colon and rectum. The detection of solitary or a few isolated lesions in the lungs should be aggressively treated surgically. A solitary shadow in the lung of a patient with cancer of the colon may be a sign of a primary or secondary lesion, and every effort should be made to achieve the correct diagnosis and institute proper management (14).

Barium Enema

The double-contrast barium enema is helpful in detecting anastamotic recurrences and new colonic lesions. It should be given at the end of one year, and subsequently every two to three years, following curative resections. The preparation for the examination should be vigorous; the patient should drink castor oil and milk of magnesia and take tap-water enemas.

Colonoscopy

Since there is a high incidence of adenomas in patients with cancer, the colon should be completely investigated by colonoscopy, preferably before surgery, but if colonoscopy is not feasible, the procedure should be done six months after surgery and probably should be repeated once every three years, in conjunction with a barium enema.

FOLLOW-UP OF PATIENTS WITH ADENOMA

When an adenomatous polyp is found, an effort should be made to rule out the presence of other polyps in the colon by an air-contrast barium enema and colonoscopy. If the patient is being operated on for polyps or carcinoma, colotomy and coloscopy may also be used. The significance of this procedure lies in the fact that up to 50% of patients with a known polyp can harbor additional polyps, and 33% of patients with cancer may have a polyp at another site (15). After the colon and rectum have been cleared of any polyps to the best of the surgeon's ability, the patient's progress should be followed continously in an effort to detect new polyp formation. We believe that adenomas have the potential to become malignant; therefore, they should be removed. The incidence of the development of metachronous adenomas varies between 20 and 40%, according to some reports (16,17). That is why follow-up is very important.

The follow-up for such patients should consist of half-yearly visits, during which a sigmoidoscopy and hemoccult slides are done. A barium enema should be done every two to three years, alternating, or in conjunction with, colonoscopy.

FOLLOW-UP OF PATIENTS WITH FAMILIAL POLYPOSIS COLI

This is a hereditary disease that is transmitted as a dominant character on a single gene; it affects each generation. It is characterized by the occurrence of numerous adenomas arising from the colonic mucosa, and it is well known that these adenomas can progress to cancer. In fact, almost all patients with this disease, if left untreated, will develop colon cancer (18). Because of this predictable outcome, there is more awareness among treating physicians that such patients should undergo a colectomy to prevent the occurrence of cancer. Some patients develop desmoid tumors and bony cysts, a condition known as Gardner's syndrome.

The follow-up for these patients depends on whether there was cancer in the colon and/or whether the rectum was retained. For, in the latter instance, very close surveillance is indicated to keep the polyps under control by repeated snare removal or fulgurations and for early cancer detection. Such patients should be seen frequently until all the polyps are cleared, and then once every six months. If the colectomy was done for a colonic cancer, the guidelines for follow-up of the patient with cancer apply here as well.

REFERENCES

1. Attiyeh FF, Wanebo HJ, Stearns MW Jr: Hepatic resection for metastasis from colorectal cancer. *Dis Colon Rectum* 21:160, 1978.
2. Attiyeh FF, McCormack PM: Resected lung metastasis from colorectal cancer. *Dis Colon Rectum* (in press).
3. Riddell RH, Levin B: Ultrastructure of the "transitional" mucosa adjacent to large bowel carcinoma. *Cancer* 40:2509, 1977.
4. Weir JA: Colorectal cancer: Metachronous and other associated neoplasms. *Dis Colon Rectum* 18(1):4, 1975.
5. Whiteley HW, unpublished data.
6. Isa SS, Attiyeh FF, Quan SHQ: Double primary carcinoma of large bowel and breast. *MSKCC Clin Bull,* in press.
7. Cahan WG, Castro EB, Hajdu SI: The significance of a solitary lung shadow in patients with colon carcinoma. *Cancer* 33(2):414, 1974.
8. Winawer SJ, Miller DG, Schottenfeld D, et al: Feasibility of fecal occult blood testing for detection of colorectal neoplasia. *Cancer* 40(5):2616, 1977.
9. Booth SN, Jamieson GC, King JPG, et al: Carcinoembryonic antigen in management of colorectal carcinoma. *Br Med J* 4:183, 1974.
10. Mackay AM, Patel S, Carter S, et al: Role of serial plasma C.E.A. assays in detection of recurrent and metastatic colorectal carcinomas. *Br Med J* 4:382, 1974.
11. Martin EW, James KK, Hurtubise PE, et al: The use of C.E.A. as an early indicator for gastrointestinal tumor recurrence and second-look procedures. *Cancer* 39(2):440, 1977.
12. Wanebo HJ, Stearns MW, Schwartz MK: Use of C.E.A. as an indicator of early recurrence and as a guide to a selected second-look procedure in patients with colorectal cancer. *Ann Surg* 188(4):481, 1978.
13. Minton JP, Martin EW: The use of serial C.E.A. determinations to predict recurrence of colon cancer and when to do a second-look operation. *Cancer* 42(3):1422, 1978.
14. Cahan WG: Multiple primary cancers, one of which is lung. *Surg Clinics North America* 49(2):323, 1969.
15. Deddish MR, Hertz RE: Colotomy and coloscopy in the management of neoplasms of the colon. *Dis Colon Rectum* 2(1):133, 1959.
16. Ekelund GR, Norden JG, Wenkert A, et al: Metachronous colorectal polyps. *Dis Colon Rectum* 17:116, 1974.
17. Kirsner JB, Moeller HC, Palmer WL, and Gold SS: Polyps of the colon and rectum—statistical analysis of a long term follow-up study. *Gastroenterology* 39:178, 1960.
18. Bussey HJR: *Familial Polyposis Coli.* Baltimore, MD, The John Hopkins University Press, 1975.

Index